Dying to be Men

Young men are on the front lines of civil unrest, riots and gang warfare worldwide. In countries such as Jamaica, Brazil, Colombia and South Africa, young men are dying at rates higher than in countries with declared wars, and at rates that are far higher than young women and older men. The principal causes of death for these young men are violence, traffic accidents and HIV/AIDS. Because they are trying to live up to certain rigid models of what it means to be men they are, literally, dying to be men.

This book looks at the challenges that young men face when trying to grow up in societies where violence is prevalent. It describes the young men's struggles in other areas of their lives, such as the effort to stay in school, the multiple challenges of coming of age as men in the face of social exclusion, including finding meaningful employment, their interactions with young women, their sexual behaviour and the implications of this for HIV/AIDS prevention. The text ultimately focuses on 'voices of resistance' – young men who find ways to stay out of violence and to show respect and equality in their relationships, even in settings where male violence and rigid attitudes about manhood are commonplace.

Dying to be Men traces the challenges facing young men in a variety of low-income urban settings worldwide and is one of the first comparative reflections of its kind. It will be invaluable reading for students and researchers of gender studies as well as practitioners working with youth, as it adds the voices of low-income young men; it also brings a gender component to the discussion of violence and delinquency, social exclusion and young people's health.

Gary T. Barker is Chief Executive of Instituto Promundo – an NGO based in Rio de Janeiro, Brazil, working in gender equality, violence prevention, HIV/AIDS and youth development. He has coordinated research and programme development on the socialization of young men in Latin America, the Caribbean, Africa, Asia and North America, in collaboration with international and national organizations. This book is based on nearly ten years of field work with young men in Brazil, the Caribbean, the United States and parts of sub-Saharan Africa, including the author's direct work with young men in these settings in collaboration with governments and NGOs.

gender studies/social studies/youth studies/health studies/delinquency/HIV/Aids

Sexuality, Culture and Health series

Edited by
Peter Aggleton, Institute of Education, University of London, UK
Richard Parker, Columbia University, New York, USA
Sonia Correa, ABIA, Rio de Janeiro, Brazil
Gary Dowsett, La Trobe University, Melbourne, Australia
Shirley Lindenbaum, City University of New York, USA

This new series of books offers cutting-edge analysis, current theoretical perspectives and up to the minute ideas concerning the interface between sexuality, public health, human rights, culture and social development. It adopts a global and interdisciplinary perspective in which the needs of poorer countries are given equal status to those of richer nations. The books are written with a broad range of readers in mind, and will be invaluable to students, academics and those working in policy and practice. The series also aims to serve as a spur to practical action in an increasingly globalised world.

Dying to be Men

Youth, masculinity and social exclusion

Gary T. Barker

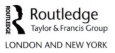
Routledge
Taylor & Francis Group

LONDON AND NEW YORK

First published 2005 by Routledge
2 Park Square, Milton Park, Abingdon, Oxon, OX14 4RN

Simultaneously published in the USA and Canada
by Taylor & Francis Inc
29 West 35th Street, New York, NY 10001

Routledge is an imprint of the Taylor & Francis Group

© 2005 Gary T. Barker

Typeset in Sabon by J&L Composition, Filey, North Yorkshire
Printed and bound in Great Britain by Cromwell Press, Trowbridge,
Wiltshire

British Library Cataloguing in Publication Data
A catalogue record for this book is available from the British Library

Library of Congress Cataloguing in Publication Data
A catalog record for this book has been requested

ISBN 0-415-33774-7 (hbk)
ISBN 0-415-33775-5 (pbk)

Contents

Acknowledgements   vi
Abbreviations   viii

1 Why the worry about young men?   1

2 'Are you a hippy or a kicker?': a personal story and a way of
   understanding manhood   12

3 'Don't worry, I'm not a thief': the story of João   26

4 The trouble with young men: coming of age in social exclusion   41

5 In the headlines: interpersonal violence and gang involvement   59

6 No place at school: low-income young men and educational
   attainment   84

7 'If you don't work, you have to steal': low-income
   young men and employment   102

8 In the heat of the moment: relating to women, having sex   117

9 Learning to live with women, becoming fathers   134

10 Dying to be men, living as men: conclusions and final
   reflections   145

Appendix   158
Notes   170
References   174
Index   181

Acknowledgements

I am able to tell these stories and attempt to make some sense of them only because young men have agreed to talk to me and tell me their stories, and because men and women who worked with these young men assisted me in this process. For the fieldwork in Brazil, I owe tremendous gratitude to Luiz dos Santos, Marcos Nascimento and Marcio Segundo; in Chicago to Sherwen Moore; and in Nigeria, to Christine Ricardo and Mohamed Yahaya.

The research presented in this book was funded by several sources, including an International Fellowship at the Chapin Hall Center for Children at the University of Chicago and an Individual Projects Fellowship from the Open Society Institute. Portions of the research were also funded by the John D. and Catherine T. MacArthur Foundation, by the Horizons Program (funded by the US Agency for International Development and administered by Population Council and partners), the World Health Organization/Pan American Health Organization, Durex Condoms/SSL International, the United Nations Office on Drugs and Crime (in the case of research in the Caribbean) and the World Bank (in the case of Nigeria, Uganda and South Africa).

Numerous individuals provided support along the way. Robert Halpern, Aisha Ray, Fran Stott at the Erikson Institute for Advanced Studies in Child Development, Chicago, and Carol Harding, Loyola University-Chicago, provided insights and guidance on research design and data analysis. Miguel Fontes and Cecilia Studart of JohnSnowBrazil, and Marcos Nascimento, Marcio Segundo and Christine Ricardo at the Instituto Promundo in Brazil, where I work, provided constant moral support, research assistance and insights. Julie Pulerwitz with the Horizons Program, PATH, has served as co-principal investigator with me on the GEM Scale impact study and contributed substantially to many of the concepts included here.

Several individuals served as advisers at various moments along the way, including Harold Richman at Chapin Hall and Peter Aggleton, Institute of Education, University of London, who was indispensable as adviser to this book. Thanks to Vania Quintanilha, Luis Geronimo Farias, Veronica Barbosa and Diana Farias for administrative support, and Sonbol Shahid-Salles for research support.

I am grateful to numerous other individuals who assisted, contributed, commented, collaborated and otherwise gave of themselves to make this research possible or supported or inspired me along the way, and in general contributed to my thinking about men, gender and social exclusion. These include Benno de Keijzer, Jorge Lyra, Benedito Medrado, Michael Kaufman, Irene Loewenstein, Paul Bloem, Matilde Maddaleno, Margareth Arilha, Meg Greene, Judith Helzner, Dean Peacock, Manisha Mehta, Guilherme Dantas, Michael Kimmel, Irene Rizzini, Fernando Acosta and Maria Correia. Suyanna Linhales Barker helped all along the way and was my most constant supporter, loving critic and travel companion and more than anyone else contributed to my understanding of Rio de Janeiro's *favelas*. Thanks also to Michael Little, Ignacia Arruabarrena and Joaquin de Paul of Dartington-International, for providing a temporary research base during part of this writing.

Finally, I wish to acknowledge and thank the young men I have interviewed and worked with in Brazil, the United States, Nigeria, Uganda and the Caribbean. While they are anonymous here, their voices are felt throughout this book. Their energy and belief in peace and being a different kind of man is felt in their communities, and beyond.

For Suy, for the journeys and back again.

Abbreviations

AIDS	Acquired Immune Deficiency Syndrome
ANC	African National Congress
CIEP	Centro Integrado de Educação Primaria (Integrated Center for Primary Education)
CESPI	Centro de Estudos e Pesquisas sobre a Infância
DJ	disk jockey
ECOS	Communiçacão em Sexualidade
GEM Scale	Gender-Equitable Men Scale
HIV	Human Immunodeficiency Virus
IBGE	Instituto Brasileiro de Geografia e Estatistica (Brazilian Institute for Geography and Statistics)
ILO	International Labour Office
NCOFF	National Center on Fathers and Families
NGO	non-governmental organization
PAHO	Pan American Health Organization
STIs	sexually transmitted infections
UN	United Nations
UNAIDS	The Joint United Nations Programme on HIV/AIDS
UNESCO	United Nations Educational, Scientific and Cultural Organization
UNFPA	United Nations Population Fund
UNICEF	United Nations Children's Fund
UNODC	United Nations Office on Drugs and Crime
USU	Universidade Santa Ursula
WHO	World Health Organization

Chapter 1

Why the worry about young men?

Young men aged 15–24 die at rates far higher than their female counterparts, and at rates higher than men of any other age group. Worldwide, the leading causes of death for young men aged 15–24 are traffic accidents and homicide – both directly related to how boys and men are socialized. In much of Latin America, the Caribbean and parts of sub-Saharan Africa, the leading cause of early death far and away is homicide. Even in parts of the world where young men's mortality rates are lower overall – such as Western Europe – more than 60 per cent of mortality among boys and young men from birth to age 24 is due to external causes, again mostly accidents and violence. In countries such as Jamaica, Brazil, Colombia and some parts of sub-Saharan Africa, young men's mortality rates are higher than in countries with declared wars.

In India and other parts of South Asia, there have been numerous studies and reports on 'missing women and girls', referring to girls who were not born because of selective abortion and others who died in infancy because of the widespread bias in favour of boys. In parts of Latin America, while on a much smaller scale, there are 'missing young men'. In Brazil, for example, the 2000 census confirmed that there were nearly 200,000 fewer men than women in the age range 15–29 because of higher rates of mortality through accidents, homicide and suicide among young men (Instituto Brasileiro de Geografia e Estatistica (IBGE) 2004). By the year 2050, Brazil will have 6 million fewer men than women, principally because of violence (O Globo 2004c).

Generally, biology provides for slightly more boys to be born because the XY chromosome structure leaves boys more vulnerable to some illnesses. Nature compensates to even out the chances that there will be equal numbers of boys and girls. In some parts of the world, however, cultures intervene in gendered ways to change these ratios. In India and other parts of South Asia, the bias in favour of boys means that millions of girls are missing – they were never born or died early because of selective abortion and female infanticide. In parts of Latin America, young men are missing because they died in violence and traffic accidents: victims too, of rigid ways of defining what it means to be men and women.

In much of the world, young men die earlier than young women and die more often than older men largely because they are trying to live up to certain models of manhood – they are dying to prove that they are 'real men'. They are driving a car or motorcycle too fast mostly to demonstrate to others that they like the thrill of risk and daring. Or they are on the streets, often working, or maybe just hanging out in public spaces where gang-related and other forms of violence most frequently occur, or they gravitate to a violent version of manhood associated with gangs.

In many low-income urban areas, gangs (most involved in drug trafficking or other illegal activities) vie for territory and for the energy, loyalties and identities of young men. In some low-income areas – the garrison communities of Kingston, Jamaica, the low-income, urban areas (*comunas*) of Medellín, Colombia, Rio de Janeiro's *favelas* (low-income areas), inner city areas in the United States, and shantytowns in parts of Central and South America–gang leaders are seen by many young people as homegrown heroes.

In parts of Africa, local militia leaders and local gangs hold similar power. In the Delta region of Nigeria, armed groups of young men used to attack only foreign oil company installations and staff. In some cities, they have now extended their violence to control entire neighbourhoods. In South Africa, there are reports of former African National Congress (ANC) combatants – lacking jobs, job skills and the social recognition they once had – being involved in gang-related violence. All of these groups attract mostly low-income young men to versions of manhood who use violence as a means to cope with their sense of social exclusion.

In many such settings, gang-involved young men are sought after as sexual partners by young women and emulated by other young men. They hold power, have money in their pockets and, by their willingness to use violence against police and rival gangs, they have status. To be a *bandido* (member of the drug-trafficking group or *comando*) in Brazil's *favelas*, a drug Don in a Kingston garrison community or a *gangbanger* in a US inner city area, is to have a name and clout in a setting where many young people perceive themselves to be excluded and disenfranchised.

The violence that young men are too often victims of (and that some carry out) also has major implications for the health and well-being of girls and women. Studies from around the world find that between one-fifth and one-half of adult women surveyed have been victims of physical violence from male partners. We know that the patterns of attitudes and behaviours that lead some men to use violence against women begin in childhood and adolescence, and that this gender-based violence often begins in dating or courtship relationships.

From a public health perspective, it could be concluded from even the most superficial glance at the data that being a young man between the ages of 15 and 24, particularly a low-income, urban-based young man, is in itself a risk factor. As a researcher in Rio de Janeiro has described it, the high rate of homicides there is a 'male social pathology' (O Globo 2002a). Similarly, the World Health Organization (WHO) suggests that being male, with regard to homicide, is a 'strong demographic risk factor' (WHO 2002: 25). This clarifies the issue about as much as saying that driving a car puts one at risk for traffic accidents. To say that being a young man is a 'risk factor' or that violence in the region is a 'male social pathology' offers relatively little explanation of the factors at play. What specifically is it about being a young man, and being a low-income young man in particular, that is the risk or the pathology? And, what is known about the young men in these settings who are not involved in gang-related and other forms of violence? Indeed, how do we explain how even in low-income, violent settings, the majority of young men generally do *not* become involved in gang-related violence?

In the school setting, it has clearly been seen how rigid views about gender affect both boys and girls. Since the early 1980s, efforts to improve school enrolment in developing countries have rightly focused on the major disadvantages affecting girls and young women. As a result of these initiatives, girls' enrolment in primary education in developing countries increased from 93 per cent in 1990 to 96 per cent in 1999. According to figures by the United Nations Educational, Scientific and Cultural Organization (UNESCO 2002), 86 countries have already achieved gender parity in primary education and 35 are close to doing so. Since the early 1990s, in parts of Latin America and the Caribbean, and in a few countries in Asia, and in nearly all of Western Europe and North America, girls have been enrolled at slightly higher rates than boys and are performing better than boys in school on several measures (reading levels and standardized test scores) (UNESCO 2002). Researchers have noted that low-income, urban-based boys in some countries are the group most likely to drop out of school.

According to the United Nations Population Fund (UNFPA 2003), half of all new human immunodeficiency virus (HIV) cases occur among young people aged 15–24. Worldwide, on average young men generally have penetrative sex earlier and with more partners before forming a stable union than do young women. The exceptions are parts of sub-Saharan Africa and the Caribbean, where girls have earlier average ages of sexual debut, sometimes as a result of forced or coerced sex by older men. Boys and young men are often socialized to see themselves as having a greater need for sex, and for risky sex, and as sexually dominating women. Even after forming stable unions or getting married, men are also more likely than women to have occasional sexual partners outside their stable relationship. This greater number of sexual partners and longer period of sexual experimentation stage for young men on average than young women has major implications for HIV transmission, and is another rationale for seeking to understand their needs and realities and directing services and education to them.

Violence in major cities may be a male social pathology. By the same token, HIV and the acquired immune deficiency syndrome (AIDS) is largely spread by the sexual behaviour of men, whether with male or female partners. The majority of cases of HIV/AIDS in the world occur via sexual transmission between men and women. Approximately one in every seven cases of HIV infection worldwide is via sexual transmission between men. An estimated 10 per cent of the world's cases of HIV are via injecting drug use; 80 per cent of those among men (Panos Institute 1998). In sub-Saharan Africa, the vast majority of HIV transmission is heterosexual, often in situations in which men's greater power in intimate relationships means that they control or dominate sexual decision-making. We might also say then that HIV, in the way it is spread, is mostly a function of the sexual behaviour of men. While the number of women who are HIV-positive is now higher than men in some countries, it is the sexual behaviour of men that largely drives the epidemic.

Recognizing these trends, in 2000–01, the Joint United Nations Programme on HIV/AIDS (UNAIDS) dedicated its World AIDS Campaign to the issue of men's behaviour and the transmission of HIV/AIDS. Background documents for the campaign sought to place men's sexual behaviour in a context of gender socialization, explaining how the way boys and men are raised in many parts of the world makes both them and their partners vulnerable to HIV/AIDS. Nonetheless, in some parts of the world, the tendency has been to blame men for HIV/AIDS. A headline in a newspaper in Portugal, reacting to the campaign, said: 'AIDS: Men are to blame' (A Capital 2000).

In 2003, with the Global Emergency AIDS Act in the US Congress, some lawmakers in the United States decided that African men were the problem behind HIV/AIDS and included language in the bill that called for changing how African men treat women, with funding provided for 'assistance for the purpose of encouraging men to be responsible in their sexual behavior, child rearing and to respect women'. While many persons would likely agree with the sentiment of this statement, it is important that we avoid blaming individual men and instead examine more closely how it is that social constructions of gender and manhood lead to HIV-related vulnerability.

Indeed, in the name of thoughtful inquiry, policy development and social justice, it is imperative to understand what exactly it is about the socialization of some men and boys that leads to these behaviours. Simply blaming men and boys leads to punitive, unjust and ineffective policies. In many parts of the world, it has become something of a national sport to demonize young men, particularly low-income young men – and in Brazil and the United States, low-income young men of African descent or other immigrant groups. Punitive policies and widespread incarceration, as opposed to genuine rehabilitation and reinsertion programmes, are the norm in Latin America, much of the English-speaking Caribbean and the United States. In the United States and Brazil, as has been widely reported, young men of African American descent are far more likely to have been in prison than to have studied in university. In one neighbourhood in Rio de Janeiro, Brazil, among 450 men interviewed, aged 15–60, 29 per cent had been arrested or picked up by police at least once.[1]

As French sociologist Loïc Wacquant (2001) and other authors have argued, zero tolerance policies, whether in Brazil, the United States or the United Kingdom have resulted in the rounding up of large numbers of young people, usually low-income young men (and often from disadvantaged immigrant groups or those of African descent), or the incarceration of these young men over relatively minor offences. It has become convenient in some policy-making circles in parts of the world to incarcerate low-income young men rather than to try to understand how delinquent behaviour might be prevented, or to understand the contexts of structural disadvantage, life circumstances and gender socialization that lead to such behaviours.

Some authors have suggested that too many young men in a society is a problem and that the age structure of many developing countries – of having too many idle and unemployed young men – is in itself a factor associated with violence. For example, a World Bank document states: 'Large-scale unemployment, combined with rapid demographic growth, creates a large pool of idle young men with few prospects and little to lose' (Michailof et al. 2002: 3). Clearly, unemployment is a major issue for economies with rapid population growth and a large population of youth seeking work.

Various researchers describe out-of-work young men as a menace and in negative and pessimistic tones, with the implication that they can and will be sucked into violence at any moment. Mesquida and Wiener (1999) make a strong and convincing case that one of the most reliable factors in explaining conflict is the relative number of young men compared to the population as a whole. They attribute young men's violence to competition for female partners and competition with older males for access to economic and political resources. In analysing data from more than 45 countries and 12 tribal societies, they find – even controlling for income distribution and per capita gross national product, which themselves are also associated with conflict – that the ratio of young men aged 15–29 for every 100 men aged 30 and over is associated with higher rates of conflict. In a similar vein, Cincotta et al. (2003) state:

> Why are youth bulges so often volatile? The short answer is: too many young men with not enough to do. When a population as a whole is growing, ever larger numbers of young males come of age each year, ready for work, in search of respect from their male peers and elders. Typically, they are eager to achieve an identity, assert their independence and impress young females. While unemployment rates tend to be high in development countries, unemployment among young adult males is usually from three to five times as high as adult's rates, with lengthy periods between the end of schooling and first placement in a job.
>
> (Cincotta et al. 2003: 44)

Other authors have argued, however, that having a large population of young men is not sufficient to explain the kind of violence and conflict that occur, nor the intricacies with how specific violent groups form and how youth do or do not become part of such groups (see Urdal 2002, for example). Indeed, however compelling the argument is that too many young men is the problem, it is important to affirm that in any of these settings, only a minority of young men participate in such conflicts. For example, the vast majority of young men – even those unemployed and out-of-school – were not involved in Charles Taylor's war in Liberia, nor become involved in gangs in Rio de Janeiro's *favelas*. Indeed, even in the poorest countries with the largest proportion of youth in their populations, the vast majority of young men do not get involved in violence. There is tremendous variation within countries and among young men, and numerous intervening variables from family to community, to individual perceptions. In many settings, there is ultimately a racist implication in such arguments that low-income young men (many of whom are of African descent) in places like Africa are inherently violent and unstable for societies.

Thus, to associate violence or the spread of HIV/AIDS with manhood or masculinities, or too many young men in a society is necessary, but not sufficient. Violence is nearly always gendered, as it also takes place within specific dimensions and conditions of power, social class structure and cultural context, as are the behaviours and circumstances that facilitate the transmission of HIV/AIDS. But it must be kept in mind that serious interpersonal violence is carried out only by a minority of young men, even in the low-income settings discussed here. And, interpersonal violence is only one issue related to low-income young men, as is HIV/AIDS.

Another caveat is in order. Fundamentally, these overall tendencies related to violence, HIV/AIDS and education mask the tremendous diversity of young men and their realities. For every young man who recreates traditional and sometimes violent versions of manhood, there is another young man who lives in fear of this violence. For every young man who hits his female partner, there is a brother or son who cringes at the violence he witnesses men using against his sister or his mother. For every young man who refuses to use a condom, there is another who discusses sexual health issues with his partner. In discussions of male 'social pathologies', particularly in discussions related to HIV/AIDS and to violence, these alternative voices are often lost.

These issues must also be understood within the context of social exclusion. As will be discussed, the needs, realities and socialization of young men and young women in southern countries, and in low-income areas in northern, more industrialized countries, take place against a backdrop of unequal access to education, employment and income. At the same time, these young men live in consumer-oriented economies in which young people are the deliberate targets of mass marketers. In this skewed system, low-income young people too often lack legitimate means to acquire those very goods they are bombarded into wanting.

This book will ask: what is the trouble with young men? It is impossible to answer that question without also looking at the underlying perversity of social structures that measure individual worth and status by goods acquired and consumed, that target a steady stream of messages to young men and young women to want certain goods, to dress certain ways, and then deprive them of the means to acquire those goods.

Behind all of these issues, culturally proscribed versions of manhood, of what societies and individuals define what it means to be a man, are at play. Researchers and advocates for more than 30 years have created a field of 'gender studies' and carried out gender analyses examining how culturally proscribed versions of womanhood – of what it means to be a woman – have constrained and limited the life choices, health and well-being, and human rights of girls and women. These studies and initiatives opened the door for seeing gender as a social – not a biological – phenomenon, and for understanding how some aspects of manhoods as traditionally constructed are often harmful or negative for women and girls.

More recently, newer questions in the field of gender studies have emerged. Women and men have recognized that there are often negative consequences for men and boys in some of the ways that manhoods are traditionally and rigidly constructed in many parts of the world. A partial list of some of these negative outcomes has already been presented: dying younger, driving too fast, using violence to achieve their ends and dropping out of school earlier in part because of having to work outside the home at relatively early ages. All of these will be discussed in detail.

At times the field of gender studies or gender has been polarized: girls and women are always dominated and subjugated and men and boys are always dominant, brutish and obtain benefits from the unequal gender order, what Australian sociologist R.W. Connell (1994) has called the 'patriarchal dividend'. Some voices in the field have said that until the inequalities affecting girls and women are redressed, that the issues of boys and men are secondary. Most advocates and researchers, however, are now saying that women's well-being cannot be improved without including boys and men and that it is vital to examine how some narrowly and rigidly defined versions of masculinity also bring with them negative consequences for boys and men.

In saying this, however, we must be careful not to throw out, or portray as negative, all gendered and sexed aspects of being human. The specific and different ways that young women and young men experience sexual pleasure, for example, are not inherently bad and should not be characterized as such. The problem arises when domination, coercion or power imbalances exist, or when one gendered or sexed way is portrayed as better or superior to the other. The gendered pleasure that boys experience in testing the limits of their physical strength and stamina can be positive – and is a realm that is increasingly being opened up for girls and women. The pleasure that many women derive from breastfeeding is positive; the problem is when women are reduced to maternal roles or subjugated. Again, the challenge is how to open the realm of caregiving in all its forms to boys and men. Men will not be able to breastfeed – without considerable biomedical re-engineering – but they can and should take on caregiving roles. This is all to say that sex differences and gender differences are not inherently bad; it is power imbalances and rigidly proscribed gender differences that are the problems.

This book emerges from the perspective that narrowly defined gender orders are negative for boys, girls, men and women. It will explore the realities, complexities and vulnerabilities of low-income, urban-based young men across several domains of their health and development. This book will rely heavily on the words and experiences of young men interviewed since 1994 in the United States and Brazil, and to a lesser extent in the Caribbean and Nigeria, and other parts of Africa. It will rely most heavily on interviews with young men in Brazil, where I live, to provide in-depth examples and case studies. It will be impossible in this space to do justice to the complexity of the cultural and contextual differences between young men in these four settings, but comparisons and differences will be highlighted. For example, the dimension of race, or ethnicity, and social exclusion based on race is a major factor in the United States, Brazil and the Caribbean for the young men interviewed there – nearly all of whom were of African descent in those three settings. In Nigeria and Uganda, for example, race is a 'constant', but social class differences and religious and ethnic group tensions loom large for low-income young men, intersecting with what it means to be a man. In sum, in including so many regions, we will lose in-depth detail but be able to demonstrate that these trends and issues – of boys dying to be men – are not an isolated phenomenon.

This book will examine five major issues related to young men in these settings:

- the general challenges they face to coming of age in settings of social exclusion
- their vulnerability to becoming involved in gang-related violence or being a victim of such violence
- their gender-specific access to and performance in school
- their access to the job market, the challenges they face in acquiring employment and the meaning of work in terms of defining their identities
- their interactions with young women, including becoming fathers and issues related to sexuality and reproductive health as well as the use of violence in intimate relationships, and the implications of these for HIV/AIDS prevention.

This book will focus mostly on young men who define themselves as heterosexual, or on heterosexual masculinities. It will comment on the homophobic attitudes of some young men, and on the role of homophobia in socializing young men, but the focus is specifically on heterosexual young men, their attitudes toward young women, and their interactions with the violent versions of manhood associated with gang-related violence (which is also largely heterosexual and often homophobic).

The focus here is on a fairly loose population called 'young men,' referring to young people between the ages of 15 and 24. These age boundaries are not, however, fixed in stone. 'Youth' in Nigeria, for example, can go up to 30 years according to some federal government policies, and up to 40 and beyond according to how families and communities define hierarchy and power over the life-cycle.

The reasons for focusing on *young* men are multiple. Youth is a socially constructed life phase and phenomenon that is lived out within the biological matrix of puberty and adolescent physiological development – and puberty itself is lived out in the socially constructed matrix of gender. Young men experience the biological, body-based phenomena of spermarche (having the first ejaculation), sexual desire and a physical growth spurt (both in height and muscle mass) within socially proscribed frameworks that measure and assess this sexual desire, growth and stamina. Biology provides a template – the hardware – for physical growth, sexual desire and reproductive capabilities.

Society in turn creates and recreates a valorative framework for these biological phenomena and provides hierarchies. Being bigger, faster and stronger and using violence to resolve conflicts and achieve dominance are often valued or glorified, while being smaller, having a modest physical stature and modest strength and using words instead of fists to resolve conflicts frequently are not. Having more sexual conquests is valued, that is channelling sexual desire in a way that emphasizes quantity of relationships and partners rather than quality in relationships. And of course, that sexual desire and the biological phenomenon of ejaculation must be engaged in heterosexual activity (or at least fantasizing about heterosexual sex). To be a 'real man' in most settings any same-sex attraction must be repressed or denied.

Youth is also the phase of life when young men generally have their first penetrative sex, experience their first intimate relationships (not necessarily in the same relationships), and are enjoined to acquire work or earn income outside the household. It is during this period when many young men leave school or are forced out of school. Young men are crossing the socially defined space between childhood and adulthood and generally taking on more complex and demanding roles in society.

They are also becoming aware. Again, biology provides a template for neurological development – for the ability to think, reason and contemplate in abstract ways. Not all human beings achieve this potential, and not all cultures promote this kind of thinking, but the biological potential for abstract thinking is, from what we know from the field of neurosciences, universal. With abstract thinking comes the ability to imagine what-if and to compare ideals – of justice, access to goods and income, those who have and those who want – with the realities of tremendous inequalities. Young men and women can, and in some settings do, project and imagine the kind of persons they want to be – they acquire subjectivity. It is within this imagining, this self-awareness and this ability to compare ideals with the real, that psychic frustration emerges. We will hear in the voices of many young men frustration over social exclusion and over their lack of access of power and income and women and a keen awareness of their limited ability to change these realities.

Nigerian young men show anger toward the 'elites' and the *Al-hajis* (men, of some income, who have done the pilgrimage to Mecca). Youth living in post-apartheid South Africa show frustration over the lack of jobs and compare the ideal they once held of social equality coming with democracy with the reality of tremendous income inequalities. Low-income Brazilian young men show resentment toward middle class youth and adults and sometimes toward drug traffickers who they perceive get 'all the good girls'. African American young men in the United States show a similar disdain toward white young men (and whites in general) and to gangbangers. Low-income Caribbean youth compare themselves to their North American counterparts and those Caribbean young men who were able to migrate to the United States. Behind this frustration is a comparison between what they would like to achieve (or what society tells them they should achieve) and what they are able to achieve.

This frustration, apart from the psychological strain it causes on young men themselves, is the incubator of social unrest and of some forms of violence (including gang involvement), seen in various forms in the areas studied here: ethnic tensions in Nigeria, violence in the garrison communities of Jamaica and drug-trafficking gangs in the United States and Brazil. Low-income young men in these settings are frequently torn between using conventional, non-violent means to achieving their ends and acquire status, income and women (or perhaps not to be able to acquire these things), or using violent ways to achieve them, which generally involves becoming part of gangs or violent groups. As one young man in Brazil said: 'Either you're going to work, or you're going to rob. But you're not gonna be 25 years old and depending on your parents.'

This gravitation toward a violent version of manhood or a conventional, 'working man' version of manhood is perhaps the central identity struggle for young men in these settings. In all these settings, and around the world, there is a clear and direct social pressure to achieve a productive version of manhood – in some settings, by whatever means necessary. There is individual decision-making involved in this process, at least for most young men. There are others, however, who seem to merely go with the flow, following the actions of their peers or families with relatively little reflection. But even those young men who apparently choose to be part of gangs or violent versions of manhood perceive pressure and expectations to produce or earn money, even if it involves violence.

Finally, there is a demographic reason for focusing on young men aged 15–24 in 2004. The majority of the world's population lives in developing countries or southern countries. Due to fertility trends, the size of the present-day youth population (using the World Health Organization's definition of youth, ages 10–24) is larger both numerically and proportionally than it has ever been. Nearly half of the people alive now on the planet are under age 25, and 1 billion are between the ages of 10 and 19 (UNFPA 2003). With declining fertility in most of the world, there will likely never be in human history a youth cohort this large again. Pessimists, as discussed earlier, see this as cause for alarm.

Others see young men's violence or unsafe sexual activity as a passing behaviour, arguing that most boys grow out of delinquency and risk-taking behaviour, which some young men do. But this argument that youth is a passing phase, or that youth violence is a 'developmental' phenomenon that passes with age, makes sense only if we see young people as human beings in the making and not actual human beings in the present. For the young people of this generation, alive in the here and now, violence and unsafe sexual behaviour has very real consequences and those who suffer from these cannot wait around for 'youthful behaviour' to pass.

Optimists, myself included, see the current youth demographic wave as an opportunity. Rethinking gender norms together with the current youth cohort, particularly rethinking what it means to be a man, could have implications for today's youth and generations to come. Of course, changing the gender order is not straightforward or simple, nor is it mine or yours to carry out. It is complex, usually slow, and must be carried out by and with communities and young people themselves. It must be collective and it must be structural; reaching two dozen in one low-income community will not lead to broad social change. While the challenge is enormous, there are some ideas of how and where to start this kind of process.

This book is part overview, part research, highly pragmatic and at times highly personal. In my professional activities, I have taken an activist stance on these issues and I will show that mindset in this book. My burning questions are: from what is known about how young men are socialized, what can we do to change the directions of some of these trends? How can we promote versions of manhood that are less violent, more gender-equitable and better for young men and young women? What has been learned from existing experiences in engaging communities, policy-makers and young men themselves in promoting other ways of being men? This book will conclude with implications and insights on what can be done about these issues – to promote versions of manhood based on respect, non-violence and a culture of care rather than on violence and domination.

Chapter 2

'Are you a hippy or a kicker?'

A personal story and a way of understanding manhood

This book is highly personal. For those of us working and researching in the areas of social sciences, social work and social change, there is nearly always some autobiography in the themes in which we work. I have chosen the issue of young men and their vulnerabilities in part because of personal experiences in my own coming of age as a young man in the 1970s in George W. Bush's Texas. These events shaped the way that I approach these issues, which has subsequently been influenced by life experiences in Latin America (where I currently live), and in other parts of the world. That said, it is appropriate to start this book with a personal story of manhood and violence (accordingly, this chapter will make extensive use of the first person).

In 1973, my family lived in Houston, Texas, in an expanding middle-class, mostly white suburb in a city fast growing – in large part because of the booming oil industry (this is the same Houston where the Bush family was making its fortune at the time). During the school year in 1973, in an empty hallway in junior high school on my way to physical education (PE) class, two boys about my age at the time (12 years old) approached me menacingly and, each holding me by a shoulder, pushed me against the wall. They were dressed in cowboy boots, tight-fitting jeans that opened slightly at the leg to offer space for the boots, and were wearing belts with large, metal buckles (the kind George W. Bush wears when he is at his ranch).

'Are you a hippy or a kicker (cowboy)?' one of them asked, looking me in the eye.

'Umm, neither,' I answered, which was the truth and the first thing that occurred to me. I was not dressed like a kicker, and didn't hang out with these two guys nor their friends, so to say I was a kicker seemed a cop-out. By my dress and not-too-long hair they could probably see that I wasn't marking myself as a hippy.

'Which is it, hippy or kicker?' one of them asked again, this time the two of them pushing both of my shoulders into the wall.

'Kicker,' I said.

'That's better,' said one of them, and the two walked away. I continued on to my PE class, shoulders sore, but everything in place. I recall feeling relieved that no one else saw the incident.

About two years before, when I was 10, I remember having become involved in a fight with a bigger boy over a girl, this time in a very public arena. She liked me, but he was bigger and decided that he had seen her first. I ended up on the ground with a bleeding lip while a group of fellow students looked on. I didn't really even know the girl. Our only encounter had been a few words spoken when we were at an outing for her birthday. I would probably have been ashamed for her to know that I had gotten into a fight because of her. But it was not really because of her. It was because of those other boys watching: would Gary Barker wimp out, or would he fight back?

Reputations and masculine identities are made this way: by signifying to girls that you will fight to be with them or because of them, and to other boys that you will hold your own. Word would get around. Whether I fought or walked away would, in my 10-year-old boy's logic, determine if other boys respected me and girls found me interesting.

This time, though, with the 'kickers', I capitulated without losing too much face, and didn't have to take a punch. On an average day in a junior high school hallway in Houston, Texas, in the mid-1970s, that wasn't too bad.

Such were some of the choices of manhood in my suburban Houston high school in the early to mid-1970s. A hippy, in the eyes of the kicker, was to be wimpy, wussy, marijuana-smoking, no good at a fight, a wearer of loose jeans and long hair, and a slouch. Hippies in my high school in the 1970s would rather make out with their girlfriends by the lockers than get in a fight. A TransAm, Camaro, or any car long and sleek with tinted windows so the police couldn't see the smoke were the preferred cars. And cars were, after all, necessary for being 'real' men of any kind – hippies or cowboys – in Houston, Texas. A kicker, on the other hand, was a straight-backed, boot-wearing, short-haired guy who liked to drink beer, something that made you wiry – not laid-back like pot. The pick-up truck was the vehicle of choice, preferably with a rifle rack in the rear window.

To these versions of manhood, add the jocks (the athletes, some of whom were also kickers, some of whom liked to hang out with hippies, and some who just hung out with the jocks); nerds (Honor Society types, science-fiction book readers, and those of Asian descent); and a few free radicals who did not fit into any of those or could manage not to have to affiliate exclusively with any one group, or circulated within various of them because they were funny enough, good-looking (or had good-looking sisters that guys in any of these groups wanted to be close to). I was in drama class, the creative writing society, the Honor Society and the tennis team, which might have made me nerd material, if not an outright wimp.

I tried on the jock identity for a short time, though, in my 'real man' career. For one year, I tried out for and made the football team (that is the

US version with shoulder pads and helmets), which was the sport for 'real' men. It was the rite of passage to the most glorified version of manhood around, that of the star athlete. I was on the B squad, the second-best squad. I endured the taunts of a coach who frequently told us that his grandmother was faster, stronger and more of a man than any of us. There was a short-lived thrill in putting on the gear, running onto the field and hearing the cheers from the drill squad (the pom-pom girls), even if they too were the B squad cheerleaders. They were not the most talented and attractive cheerleaders and we were not the best football players – but we were all trying to fit into the gender ideals.

These were important issues in adolescent, and male adolescent development – and still are in many parts of the world. Namely, who am I? Which group do I project my self or a version of self into? The Who-am-I question is partly intrapsychic, but also concerns a public projection of self. More precisely, which version of adolescent manhood, or gendered adolescent identity, do I want others to see? For most of us, this public projection of manhood is often a nuisance; other times it is a farce.

But it has very real consequences. Deviation from gender norms can result in ridicule and being excluded from certain spaces (after I left the football team, for example, I was rarely invited to the jock parties). For some young men, the version of manhood internalized, projected and lived is a matter of life and death. Attacking, bashing, even killing gay young men, or transvestite young men, has become too common in some cities in Brazil and elsewhere. If we ask the bashers why they bash, they usually cannot tell us, but we can surmise: they attack those who do not live to their expectations of what men should be. We can find examples of this in various parts of the world. In contemporary Japan, there have been an increasing number of cases of out-of-work, homeless men being attacked by groups of middle class boys and young men. The motive: these homeless, 'worthless' men are an affront to the idealized Japanese version of the working man (New York Times 2003). In Brazil, where I live, there have been attacks by heterosexual middle class young men on gay men coming out of nightclubs in Rio de Janeiro. Again, the motive is attacking versions of manhood that do not match the ideal. In my middle class world, I was able to trade football for other sports, and other meaningful, socially recognized identities, and still save face, but what of those low-income young men who find no other accessible model of manhood apart from gangs?

I offer two more examples of seeing these issues in action. About three years after the hippy-kicker incident, in 1976, I was eating lunch in my high school cafeteria, along with about 200 other students, when I heard the sound of a gunshot. Firecrackers, I thought, at first. I remember thinking: someone will get expelled for this. Then, looking up, I saw two young men, near the line for food. One was pointing and firing a handgun. I heard and saw a second and then a third shot fired at the other young man, in the abdomen and chest area. Still, disbelief. Maybe they were in the drama group. Then again, I didn't know them (or at least I didn't recognize them at first) and I was in the drama club. The boy being shot fell and at that moment I saw blood. Fake blood? I wondered. He stayed on the ground and blood flowed. My classmates and I realized that this was in fact real.

There was a collective silence, then screams, followed by girls crying. The boy with the gun ran and a teacher (a PE coach, who was a former police officer) ran after him and out of the school. We were led outside into the courtyard of the school. Girls continued to cry. 'Wow, can you believe that?' the boys were saying. 'Do you know who it was?' others were asking. I recognized one of the boys (the victim); he had been in some junior high school classes with me, but he was not a friend, nor part of my social group. I knew his name but almost nothing else about him. I remember him as being a bully back in junior high. A short time later, we were escorted back to our classes. Later that afternoon, an announcement came over the loudspeaker system: 'The two boys involved in the incident in the cafeteria were not from our high school [they were from the adjacent high school]. No students from our school were involved nor harmed in the incident.'

Nothing else was officially said. Back to class. Don't forget your homework. Plans were made so that the rest of the students could have lunch elsewhere. In the hallway, the story that circulated was that the fight was over a girl. The boy who was killed (Barry) was going out with the ex-girlfriend of the boy who killed him (Ralph).[1] Ralph had got the gun out of his father's closet. And so the story ended. No counselling was offered to students who witnessed the killing nor for friends of the young men involved. There was no public grieving at school nor any official discussion of what happened and how it might be prevented. The football game the following Saturday went on as usual. The implicit message was that all was okay, that this was a random, unfortunate event, and that there was nothing particularly wrong with the way manhood was constructed. Indeed, the issue of manhood or gender was never invoked.

Now, jump ahead 15 years. I was living in Bogotá, Colombia, where I worked for an international non-governmental organization (NGO) in the area of youth development. I was at a conference on sexuality education and HIV/AIDS prevention in Medellín. It was late at night and after a long day of presentations and meetings I was nearly falling asleep in the taxi that took two colleagues and myself back to the hotel from dinner. The year was 1991 and Medellín was heavily armed; Carlos Escobar was at large and the government's reputation was at stake in capturing him. Motorcycle police, with two officers on the motorcycle, swarmed the streets and road blocks were common.

Our taxi suddenly came to a quick stop to avoid hitting a car and two police on a motorcycle, who had stopped a young man and young woman on a motorcycle. The motorcycle police had drawn their weapons and were pointing them at the young man. No one in our car, not even the taxi driver, said anything. The driver then started to pull away; it was safer to leave than to linger. As he pulled away we saw one of the motorcycle policeman fire several times on the young man; he fell to the ground, as the young woman screamed, and the police looked on, apparently making sure the victim did not move.

These two homicides were statistically typical – young men killing other young men. There were then (with similar rates for 2000) nearly 30,000 such incidents (homicides) per year in Colombia, and there are currently more than 16,000 homicides (the vast majority firearm-related) in the United States annually (Ayres 1998; National Center for Health Statistics 2003). More than 90 per cent of those homicides in Colombia and the United States are between men, and disproportionately among lower-income young men.

There could be, of course, entire books to write about either of those incidents. Who was the young man on the motorcycle in Medellín? Was he part of one of the drug cartels? Did he have a weapon? Who was the police officer who fired on him? What about Barry and Ralph (the two young men in my high school cafeteria)? What had happened to Ralph so that he reached the point of getting his father's gun and shooting Barry (and did so in front of 200 persons)? A veritable encyclopaedia could be written about the socialization of the two boys, their family situations, the specifics of the incidents themselves and the young men's access to weapons. The story of the killing in Medellín would, in turn, require an analysis of violence in Colombia, the story of the *comunas* (low-income, urban areas) where Escobar and other drug traffickers find their staff, the role of the state (and the police response), as well as the individual stories of the young man.

But in all these incidents, there is a common backdrop of masculinity, of male identity, of projecting and seeking to live up to a certain version of what it means to be a man. Why did I feel compelled to fight over a girl whom I really did not know and take on a boy who was clearly bigger than me? Why did I have to define myself as a hippy or a kicker? What do these definitions of manhood have to do with the high rates of homicides among young men?

The 'matrix' of gender

Among young men I have spoken with over the years in various settings, there is nearly always a clear sense that something is expected of you to be a *real* man. There are of course expectations of girls and women as well. The expectations of, or on, boys and men often include some pressure to perform, to achieve and to define oneself as not-female, not-homosexual and not-dependent. In some societies, as researchers from Margaret Mead (1949) onward have highlighted, these markers or signs of manhood (and womanhood) are clearly proscribed within rites of passage. In parts of

Africa, even now, when boys reach the age of 10 to 15, they are taken away from their villages and spend time with older men, being initiated into the rules of manhood. This may include tests of stamina and courage, and information or advice on how to treat women. In some countries (parts of South Africa, Kenya and elsewhere), these rites of passage also include circumcision, often in unhygienic conditions bringing risk of infection and in a few cases death.[2]

For example, in eastern Uganda (in and around the city of Mbale, near the border with Kenya), the Bigisu cultural group that dominates the region practises ritual male circumcision as part of the rite of passage to manhood. Every two years, young men roughly between the ages of 15 and 18 participate in a month-long process involving entire communities. Young men are circumcised without anaesthesia by 'surgeons' – men in the communities who have been trained by other men – to carry out the process.

Following the procedure, young men are to spend approximately one month in seclusion, healing from the process. When the month-long healing process is completed, the 'surgeon' and male family members speak with each young initiate, enjoining him to have sex with a woman in the village (provided it is not the woman he intends to marry). Through this ritualized sex, the young man is said to rid himself of 'evil spirits'. He is also urged to have 'live' sex, meaning sex without a condom.

The initiate is encouraged to get married as soon as possible and to begin childbearing shortly thereafter. In some villages, the young man may be given a hoe or other work instruments, so he can begin working on a plot of land. He is publicly acknowledged as having achieved manhood.[3]

Through the eyes of Westerners, this ritual may seem primitive, but it has parallels elsewhere in the world in being taken by male peers to have your first sex with a sex worker, having your first fist-fight (particularly over a girl), shooting a gun, or mistreating an animal or someone younger or smaller than you. The list could go on of markers of manhood around the world – all more or less equally valid or equally questionable.

These rituals nearly always play out on or in the body (of young men and others). Behind all of them, however, is the notion that boys must be toughened up to become men, to assume their roles as providers and protectors and sometimes as warriors. Enduring pain or inflicting pain – or both – are often part of this toughening up. Those like my 'kicker' colleagues who pushed me against the wall were themselves subjected to the process, and the pain, and in turn carry out the rituals on the bodies and psyches of the next generation of boys – and so on.

Most of the world, however, has less clear rites of passage to manhood than the Gisu, but most boys and men can read the 'code' behind the wall, or are at least aware of expectations of them – some of which are perceived as being onerous. Anthropologists and sociologists have called this code various things, and analysed it in great detail in other works. This 'code' is at times referred to as gender structure, gender hierarchies, the 'mandates of masculinity (or gender)', gender roles and social norms. The French sociologist Pierre Bourdieu (1999) called it a *habitus*; others have called it a social habitus. Harvard-based psychologist William Pollack, writing about young men in the United States, calls it the 'boys' code', which he defines as:

> a set of behaviors, rules of conduct, cultural shibboleths, and even a lexicon, that is inculcated into boys by our society – from the very beginning of a boy's life. In effect we hold up a mirror to our boys that reflects back a distorted and outmoded image of the ideal boy – an image that our boys feel under great pressure to emulate.
>
> (Pollack 1998: xxiii)

While these definitions and concepts vary, sometimes in important theoretical ways, which we will not go into here, behind them all is the notion of a social metastructure that operates via cultural practices, language, styles of living and interacting, and power distribution to promote specific ways of being men and women. Most of the time, this social metastructure operates in subtle and sometimes unperceived ways. Children and adults in many parts of the world often take the code as immutable reality. Biological sex differences are confused with or used to justify socially constructed gender differences. Men are this way, women that – and so the world goes.

At the risk of oversimplifying what is a complex social phenomenon, there is a relevant metaphor in the Wachowski Brothers' movie *The Matrix* (1999). Like the computer matrix in which the film's characters live their lives (in the film, all but a few individuals are unaware they are living in a computer matrix), gender norms form a matrix that influences human relationships and interactions, and which for many persons is unperceived. Most young men can tell us about and can perceive the social pressures to act and behave in certain ways. But most young men do not have the ability to see beyond the matrix or to see the gender matrix for what it truly is – a socially constructed set of mandates shaped and created by individuals, social structures and historical and local contexts.

Such norms are instead perceived as absolute, or related to anatomical and biological differences between men and women. Talk show hosts and pop psychology books adore this simplicity: if only women could figure out men and vice versa. There are of course gender-related tendencies; as mentioned here, men and boys are more likely to use physical violence than women and girls. But it is important to keep in mind that variation among men is greater than aggregate sex differences on every measure of gender differences. To put it simply, two men in a given setting may have less in common than they do with a woman in the same setting. If men and boys on aggregate use physical violence more that women and girls on aggregate, there are many boys who do not use violence, abhor it and are more likely to identify with how women and girls frequently react to violence.

That said, one of the main challenges to engaging young men in exploring alternative ways of being men is helping them acquire a level of metacognition – reflecting about how you think – or critical thinking to see beyond the gender matrix, to recognize it as a socially constructed phenomenon with tremendous variation and flexibility. This book will explore some of the ways this kind of critical thinking can be promoted.

What does it take to be a *real* man?

In the existing gender matrixes, what then does it take to become a man? How do cultures define manhood? Sometimes predictably and consistently, young men in Brazil, the United States, Nigeria and the Caribbean answer in common ways when asked what it means to be a man.

Showing a firm attitude or standing up for yourself is one mandate; as several young men from low-income, urban areas of Brazil said: 'To be a man is to have the right attitude', 'to hold your own', 'to stand up when you have to' and 'to defend your reputation'. This was part of the mandate that got me the bloody lip. Marking your reputation can be quite important in violent neighbourhoods. One young man in a *favela* in Rio de Janeiro said: 'being a friend [to someone] is trying to avoid fights, but if you can't avoid it, you have to defend yourself, because if not you'll just get beat up.'

Another mandate – perhaps the *key* mandate in achieving adult manhood in much of the world – is achieving some level of financial independence, employment or income, and subsequently to start a family. As another young man in Brazil said: 'To become an adult . . . move out and live on your own . . . to get a job . . . take care of your family and raise your family.' In short, you must have a job or some kind of income. Similarly, a young man in Chicago said that a boy becomes a man: 'When he don't depend on anybody and have something of his own.' Young men in Nigeria had similar responses. One said: 'When you are a boy, all the responsibility is to your parents. Then [when you become a man] you take on the bothers of your parents and from your own pocket you pay [for your things].' Another young man in Nigeria, who left school at a relatively early age and struggled to make enough money, said: 'We become men when we think about being on our own. It depends on when you get a lot of money to be free. Then you can do what you want.' The meaning of work for low-income men will be the subject of Chapter 7. In a consumer-oriented world of mass marketers who deliberately target youth, including low-income youth, this masculine mandate of working or producing income is exacerbated.

Some young men from low-income neighbourhoods in Chicago – including one neighbourhood where four out of five households were single-parent (nearly all mother-headed) households – focused on being responsible for children that they might have. Indeed, for some young men, being a responsible father was a marker of manhood: '[Being a man means] taking care of a child. I want my child to know me. I don't want my child to think that [that I abandoned him/her] about me . . . to think: "Why he leave?".' Still other young men focused on sexual conquest: 'You become a man when you have sex [with a woman].'

In all four settings described here in detail, some young men resorted to biblical or religious references about roles of men and women in society, but even in areas which might be considered highly religious, or religiously fundamental, these scriptural versions of gender and manhood are secondary or subsumed within the issue of economic independence, of being the breadwinner, and of becoming sexually active.

These examples already begin to show cultural, contextual and individual variations, which will be described in later chapters. Young men in Nigeria, for example, say they are young men up until their late twenties and even early thirties. Older men are seen as having access to women (including younger women), jobs, resources and subsequently to greater power. In Nigeria and many parts of sub-Saharan Africa, chronic poverty and disadvantage, the large youth cohort, along with hierarchical family power structures, mean that many young men seek to achieve manhood through employment but are frequently unable to do so.

For some low-income young men in Brazil, many sought to put off becoming men, partly because of the pressure this implied to acquire employment. They instead preferred to prolong the carefree time of being boys. A *real* man has to get a job – something which is not easy in such contexts. A boy has less pressure on him, at least in this setting. At the rural level in Brazil, the counterparts to these boys are pressured to work at even earlier ages. This mostly male child labour (referring specifically to labour outside the home), often in hazardous conditions, has been the subject of tremendous policy development since the early 1990s in Brazil.

This list of what it means to be a man could go on for pages, but the examples here highlight some of the major tendencies. Common to all of them (including the autobiographical examples) is a cultural mandate to prove yourself, and define which kind of man you are, and to do so in a public way. Most boys hear in their heads some cultural variation of an internalized voice saying: *Take a stand, boy!* Boys and young men often talk about an internal dialogue and struggles over this issue. Many of these boys and young men are short on words or generally utter one-word responses in the classroom setting or with their parents. But when finally asked about this internal struggle and the pressure to be a certain kind of man, their words filled up dozens of tapes and notebooks.

Two examples will be offered for illustration. One young African American man in Chicago, who was struggling to stay out of a gang and to find some version of manhood that did not involve the gangs, said this:

> [Comparing myself to other guys in school] . . . some of them don't think about responsibility. They think life is just a joke. Some of them don't know why they put on Earth . . . They try to lead me. I'm tryin' to be in the right way but right now they're leadin' me in the wrong way. . . . They led me into a gang life. Like they used to ask me if I wanted to join a gang and I really didn't want to but then I saw them havin' money and havin' clothes all the time and cars. And I said 'if they can do that, I can do that.'
>
> (Tony, 15, African American, Chicago)

Another young man in Chicago, going through a similar internal dialogue, said:

> I say, well, to me, I'm better than them [gang-involved guys in school] because I don't go around and call these girls names and actin' like I'm somethin' when I'm not or havin' to go 'round and havin' somebody to look out behind my back . . . that's what the majority of school is [these guys], gangs. You know. They say somethin' and talk they smack and then run and get their friends to help them out.
>
> (Darryl, 17, African American, Chicago)

Another young man, also in Chicago, described a daily battle to define himself as non-gang-involved. Nonetheless, even though he tried to make it clear that he did not want to be involved in gangs, gang-involved young men harassed him frequently trying to win him over to their side. His experience resembles in some ways the personal example of the hippy–kicker rivalries described at the beginning of this chapter, but the consequences are radically different between my mostly white middle class world and his mostly African American low-income neighbourhood. For this young man, being gang-involved or not could bring life-altering consequences:

> They [these guys in a gang] were approaching me, saying that I was in another gang. The gang that they was in was different, like for instance they was like Black Disciples and they was like: 'You GD' [referring to a gang called Gangster Disciples]. And I was like: 'I ain't nothing.' And they just kept on doing it. They knew I wasn't in no gang because they seen me come home with books and football equipment [but still they try to pin me on being part of a gang].

Common to all three of these examples is a conflict between a version of manhood – in this case a gang-involved version – trying to co-opt or recruit young men, and their own desires to be other kinds of men. It is ultimately an identity struggle. Identity is the public projection of a self, not necessarily a true version of self, but some version of self. As previously mentioned, common to nearly all analyses of male identities or masculinities is the public nature of having to prove one's manhood. Nearly every man I have told my hippy-versus-kicker story to (and the choice of identities in my school) has told me his. There is nearly always an array of identifiable categories of male identity you could belong to, but social settings and structures push for definition and affirmation.

Clearly as we see in these examples, some male identities have more salience or power than others, and different categories of manhood try to co-opt, to encourage other boys and young men to be like them and to obligate young men to choose an identity as they themselves were pressured to. The young man who pushed me up against the wall and wanted me to affirm that I was a kicker probably had the same done to him, or something similar. He had been raised to abhor other, *sissified* ways of being men and wanted to affirm the supremacy of his way of being a man. He may have faced a brother, father, cousin or uncle who pressured him to do something to prove he was a man (or a certain kind of man), by smoking, or getting drunk, firing a gun or chewing tobacco (which no doubt made him gag or vomit the first time he did, which probably led to feelings of superiority on the part of the other men around him, who had been humiliated in similar ways in their youth and so on).

If we are lucky, the challenges to prove our manhood result in embarrassment, a bit of shame, and perhaps public humiliation. For others, like Ralph, Barry and the young men with motorcycles and guns in Medellín, the kinds of manhood they gravitated toward or were socialized into meant death or incarceration. Ralph may have had an array of psychological and family issues, but it can be surmised that he was socialized in a setting where being a man meant not accepting shame – like the kind brought on by another boy stealing your girlfriend. In Colombia, a history of internecine fighting, social divisions and chronic fear has led in part to vendetta killing and the arming of the state and civilians. In low-income, urban and rural Colombia, too many young men are trained and hired (as part of the police, the drug traffickers and vigilante groups) to kill. But it is no statistical nor biological accident that all involved in these incidents were young men.

Framing a way of understanding young men

These personal incidents started my questioning and led to a multi-year interest and engagement as an advocate around the issues and realities of low-income young men. These experiences led me to want to understand more about the identity development process, and to offer insights on what might be done to expand the number of 'hats' (particularly healthy, positive, non-violent ones) for young men.[4]

In 1995, with a colleague, I carried out focus group discussions with 127 young men and individual interviews with ten young men aged 15–30 in conjunction with two vocational training programmes in low-income areas in Rio de Janeiro (Barker and Loewenstein 1997). Convincing staff at these two centres that it was worth using the time of young men to talk about gender and manhood was a challenge in itself. Why bother asking about the obvious? These young men need to be trained to get work, not to talk about something as vague as gender or what it means to be a man, we were told.

We heard typical and predictable stories about what it meant to them to be men: having sex and finding a job were the two main responses. It was easier to have sex, they said. In low-income Rio de Janeiro, as will be described further, finding work is the hard part. We heard a common array of homophobic comments and definitions of what men were supposed to be and do: hard workers, ready to have sex all the time, superior to women and to same-sex-attracted young men, have limited involvement in household chores, and that women deserve being hit when they disrespect men.

But in every group we spoke with there were one or two young men who publicly questioned the traditional norms. Some said, looking to the rest of the group: 'I have a friend who is gay, what's wrong with that?' Others might respond: 'Keep him with you. I don't want him to come near me.' Some young men questioned violence against women, even when the rest of the group were talking about the need for men 'to educate women' and 'keep them in line'.

In the course of this project, eight outliers were identified, what I have come to call 'voices of resistance', and we asked them back to speak with them individually. More questions were asked: How is it that you questioned the group about these things? How did that feel? How do you think you came to see these issues this way?

One young man talked about his grandmother, who after being a widow for many years, decided she wanted to begin seeing men again, and how that led him to question his ideas about gender. If his grandmother had a right to sexual agency and desire, well then, why did not all women? And, his reasoning went, if women have the same right to sexual desire as men, then they must be equal to men on other dimensions. Another young man told about having a father who worked for a European consulate. As a result of his father's work at the consulate, the young man had interacted with the consul of that country and had the chance to see how this man treated his daughters and sons equally, and perceived how as a father, the consul had equal aspirations for the professional futures of his daughters and sons.

Whether these young men acted in gender-equitable ways in their own interpersonal relationships is, of course, another question, but they did show an alternative discourse and defended their viewpoints publicly. There are also likely to have been many other young men in the group who held alternative viewpoints, but were reluctant to face the criticism of the group, or felt that being in a predominantly male setting (the vocational training schools), that they had to perform a certain kind of gender. To use the example from the beginning of this chapter, they were hippies but did not want to be pushed up against the wall by the kickers.

How many of these alternative voices or voices of resistance exist? What about parts of the world where gender roles are even more rigid than in low-income urban Brazil? Are there outliers or voices of resistance in, say, Muslim areas of Africa and Asia, or traditional rural societies? My work with young men, and the work of others, would suggest that some kind of resistance or variation can be found even in these traditional settings.

In recent discussions and interviews with young men (in school and out of school) in three cities in Nigeria, similar voices of resistance were identified. In one group discussion with Christian and Muslim young men, the prevailing discourse was that girls and women were not equal to men and that men should work, while women should care for the home and children. However, one Muslim young man stood up and said he disagreed. He said that girls and women were equal and deserved equal education and could excel in any area that men worked in (this in a part of Nigeria where Muslim leaders want to enact Sharia law). In a subsequent individual interview, the young man said he had seen in his family how women's education is important (a female cousin had her PhD). He also described how his father had used physical violence against his mother, but was reprimanded by male friends and colleagues and changed his behaviour. All these things, the young man said, had led him to change his views about girls and women.

Clearly, the factors associated with having these alternative views are more complex than this, but these were the stories these young men told about themselves and how they came to be different in terms of gender when compared to the majority of their peers. From these stories, as will be discussed in greater detail in later chapters, colleagues and I have begun discussing what can be done – at the level of policy, programme and the media – to assist more young men to acquire this critical discourse, or the ability to see through the gender matrix. The Appendix describes this research process in greater detail, along with a brief description of some of the interventions developed for engaging young men in this critical reflection.

This focus on the voices of resistance to traditional, patriarchal versions of manhood is, apart from being a useful way to approach the issue, politically important. The media and policy portrayals of young men have too often been negative. These voices of alternative views of manhood are often missing. Gang leaders make headlines; non-violent young men generally do not. We cannot, of course, whitewash the situation and pretend that all young men really are nice to women after all or that all young men are peaceful, law-abiding citizens. But it is important to pay greater attention to the variation in young men's discourses and ways of being, to understand through these voices of resistance that masculinities in these settings are not inherently violent, callous and exploitative of women. All manhoods – whether more or less violent or more or less gender-equitable – are situationally and contextually constructed. Understanding these voices of resistance yields tremendous insights on the power of subjectivity – that is the power of individuals to construct their own meaning out of the world around them and their life circumstances – particularly the power of subjectivity to question rigid gender norms.

Understanding these voices of resistance should not, however, detract from focusing on radical changes that need to be made in what it means to be a man or a woman and to providing access to education and employment for low-income youth. In the media and in the West we like stories of individual effort and overcoming the odds. These stories provide inspiration and hope and offer characters or individuals with whom we can identify. Within the field of child development, there is tremendous research devoted to the concept of resilience, which is the notion that some persons overcome the odds and endure risk and vulnerability and make something of themselves.

This approach is useful, and will sometimes be applied here, but it also has limitations. For example, based on this notion of resilience or voices of resistance, do we try to enhance the ability of young people to withstand and endure risk or vulnerability, or do we try to change the social structures and inequalities that create risk and vulnerability? Neoliberal economies typically opt for the former. True social change requires both.

In studying the identities of young men, it is imperative to keep in mind the situational nature of our identities or how we project who we are. Like others working in the field of gender, this book will use categories and labels for different versions of manhood – including, among others, violent, non-violent, more gender-equitable, patriarchal or *machista*. However, identities are fluid, changing over time and circumstance. The complexity of individuals means that these labels never fit completely, and therefore that they should be used with care.

This action-research design, with some variations, has been the same process I have pursued in various settings.[5] This approach to young men focuses on understanding the pressure to choose specific 'hats' or versions of masculinity and the power to resist that pressure to buy into a given version of manhood. It also seeks to identify factors that make it possible for some young men to acquire more gender-equitable and non-violent versions of manhood.

Paraphrasing David Byrne (from the song, 'Once in a Lifetime' by Talking Heads) I have been asking young men – particularly more gender-equitable young men and pro-social young men – to reflect on the question: 'Self, how did I get here?' How did I get to be this kind of man? How did I acquire this particular gendered identity? And from their responses, I have been working with colleagues in several countries to do something about it – at the level of policy, with the media, with communities and with young men themselves.

Chapter 3

'Don't worry, I'm not a thief'

The story of João

Why is Rio de Janeiro not more violent?

In early 2004, gang violence in Rio de Janeiro was again in the world's headlines; it was leading to deaths among police, drug-trafficking suspects and bystanders, was altering traffic patterns and was leading to pressure on policy-makers to do something – anything. Some policy-makers suggested building high walls around the *favelas* or slums to keep the violence or the *favelas* from encroaching on middle-class neighbourhoods. More enlightened voices complained of a corrupt and poorly trained police force and of the lack of opportunities for the young men involved in the drug-related violence. Eventually the military was called in to 'restore order' in one neighbourhood where violence was particularly intense.

This has been business as usual in Brazil for many years. Indeed, since at least the early 1990s, the question has frequently been asked: why is Rio de Janeiro so violent? This book will not bother to try to dispel the US State Department warnings issued, or the newspaper articles, or television news programme's 30-second news flashes, on specific incidents of violence. But a few things should be clarified. One is that the violence, specifically the fatal violence, is seldom (but sometimes) directed against the middle class. Those who should be worried about interpersonal violence are those living in low-income communities. The violence is overwhelmingly directed inward: low-income young men against other low-income young men. If you are a young man between the ages of 15 and 24, living in a *favela* in Rio, and in settings like this around the world, you should indeed be worried about interpersonal violence. A telling photo during this recent round of violence, on the front page of several newspapers in Rio and nationwide in Brazil, showed a young man, of African descent, apparently dead and face down, being carried out of the neighbourhood in a wheelbarrow. He was killed by police who said he was a drug trafficker; his family asserted that he was a working young man and father who was involved in social programmes in the community.

It is more astounding to think about the limits of the interpersonal violence in Rio de Janeiro than the extent of it. It is impressive that in the face of the social exclusion that characterizes low-income neighbourhoods in Brazil, in particular, that hordes of young men do not descend the *favelas* and start a revolution right now. Similarly, Colombia is in the midst of a contained or limited civil war, but still to walk through a low-income community in Bogotá – and compare that to the European or North American-level wealth on the north side of the city – is to wonder why the civil war is not larger than it is. The housing projects on the South Side of Chicago are not in a constant state of war, however much the middle-class media and Hollywood films may portray them as such.

Interpersonal violence happens, and happens too much in all of these places, but it is occasional violence. In the case of *favelas* and the South Side of Chicago, a gang war ensues, some reprisal killings are carried out and life returns to normal; the majority of residents, young and old, abhor this violence. But given the degree of poverty, social exclusion, unequal income distribution and racism that exists in many of these settings, it is appropriate to turn the question around: why are young men in low-income neighbourhoods in Rio de Janeiro not *more* violent than they are?

This chapter will begin to explore the dimensions of this social exclusion by looking in depth at the story of one young man and his community. What does it mean to be a young man coming of age in a setting like this? How does one deal with the pressures of achieving the mandates of manhood and at the same time struggle with social exclusion? Young men in these settings face pressure to define manhood in specific ways, but this pressure happens within the context of social exclusion. The chapter will also discuss the protective factors that keep most young men from getting involved in this violence, and the power of subjectivity to question this violence – while keeping pressure on policy-makers to make structural changes.

Policy-makers, the media, the concerned middle class (concerned with its own well-being most of the time) continue to focus on the violence of a few young men as the major issue in public safety and security. To be sure, this violence is a major human rights, public safety and public health issue. But the larger violence behind it is the structural violence that perpetuates income inequalities, classism and racism. This is the violence that underpins, frames and incubates interpersonal violence. Clearly, poverty, racism and social exclusion do not cause interpersonal violence, just as being male does not cause violence, but social exclusion is the framework for the interpersonal violence that gets the headlines.

Discussion about this structural violence is often pushed aside, or deemed too intractable, or too impolite to discuss. However, for male and female youth in low-income communities, it is *the* issue they want to discuss. Gang-related violence, educational difficulties, finding work – these too will be considered – but this analysis of young men must start with the issue most salient to them: being excluded to the margins of society.

In discussing social exclusion it is important to talk about more than just material poverty. Social exclusion means, in addition to material want, facing curtailed life and vocational options. For most low-income young men, it means being keenly aware that one is being denied access to status, goods, respect and the company of young women that could belong to them if the world were a more just place. Modern democracies in a capitalistic world offer a series of explicit and implicit promises to their populaces. One of these is the promise that if you work hard enough you will have more or less equal access to goods and status; another is equal treatment and rights. Young men are keenly aware of the promises and experience distress and frustration when they come to see these promises as false.

To discuss these issues and understand them at the level of individual young men and their communities, the story of one individual young man and his community will be examined.

A boy named João

Since 1999, I have interviewed and worked with dozens of young men from at least four different *favelas* (low-income areas) in Rio de Janeiro. All of these young men have compelling life stories and offered complex reflections on what it means to be a man in settings like this. One who stands out and whose life incidents recall the question – Why is Rio not more violent? – was a young man who will be called João.

João was 19 when he was interviewed several times for this study. He stood out among an already distinct group of young men who formed themselves into an informal clique or peer group called 'United in Peace'. Even within this group, João showed tremendous respect for women, believed in and lived an impressive degree of gender equality in his relationship with his girlfriend (and mother of their child) and was a voice for non-violence. He also had, among many young men interviewed in this setting, more than enough reasons to get involved in the drug-trafficking groups or *comandos*, to be bitter and angry toward the middle class, and the system that produces social exclusion.

João lived in a *favela* called Maré (more on Maré later), where drug-trafficking gangs were quite strong. We met him and a group of more than 20 of his peers, all young men aged 14–20, with the help of health outreach workers at the local public health clinic and teachers at the local public school. Getting the group engaged and going was a slow process. Few of the young men were accustomed to sitting still and openly conversing about issues such as violence, gender, what they wanted for their future. Most were not well-performing students, and resisted the notion of sitting still or anything that resembled a classroom. They often arrived late, talked over each other and threatened each other when one said something they did not agree with.[1]

João stood out from the start. He was on time and spoke in turn, waiting for others to finish. He rarely lost his temper. One session, he arrived with a baby in his arms and apologized to the group and the facilitators that he would not be able to participate that day because he had to take his daughter to get a vaccination.[2]

Where did this soft-spoken, polite and gentle young man come from? He came from a family where drug use and involvement in the *comandos* were high. Other personal challenges included witnessing domestic violence (his stepfather's violence against his mother), having to work on the streets at an early age, and his mother's death when he was 17. João orchestrated a temporary reunification of his father with his mother (who reunited shortly before his mother died).

One of the biggest obstacles to his life in general, schooling and search for work, was the fact that he had no birth certificate – which meant in turn that he could not get full-time work, register for obligatory military service (which in turn is an obstacle to acquiring full-time employment), legally recognize his paternity, nor enrol in formal education. The fact that he did not have a birth certificate is also an indicator of the degree of his family's disorganization during his childhood.[3] In spite of the numerous obstacles that this brought for him, he was consistently optimistic, believing that life will bring good things. He credited his grandmother with being a stable force in his life. Much of his identity and energy was invested in being an involved father for his 7-month-old daughter. He described fatherhood as something that helped him mature from a boy to a man.

João showed a positive disposition, as well as self-reflective abilities, meaning he could talk about himself, his identity and his life struggles with an impressive degree of clarity. He saw himself as different than the other boys in his seriousness and his dedication to work and to his daughter and his wife, but at the same time he was able to move back and forth between being a youth and being a 'family man':

GB: How is it for you to be father?

JOÃO: . . . it's good. A lot of people say that I messed up when I had a baby this early [he was 18 when his daughter was born]. But I say that before my girl was born, I was really in shit. I would not show up for lots of things. But when she was born, I told myself that I wasn't going to miss anything for her . . . It's good [to have a child] because I think if I hadn't of been in really good with my wife and having this baby, I think I wouldn't want anything to do with work. I would just be out having fun, dancing, going to the dances, funk dances, drinking beer. [Now] I always have to buy something for the house . . . with the money . . . I make parking cars, I'm taking care of her.

At first glance, João faces a number of life circumstances that should put him at higher vulnerability for participating in gang-related violence (the *comandos*) or substance use, including domestic violence, family separation, family substance use, family members involved in the *comandos*, low school attainment and limited vocational possibilities.

Living with social exclusion

Once, João was asked what it was like being a young man from a *favela*. He relayed an incident when he was watching and washing cars and a white, middle-class woman asked him to wash her car. When the woman returned, she claimed that he had not washed the car:

> when she came back, it [the car] was already washed but she started just saying like shit, you didn't wash it, and cussing at me. And I just stayed quiet because I knew if I started to argue, someone would call the police and pretty soon they'll be saying I'm trying to rob her. And I'm quiet, and she says: 'You didn't wash shit.' And I said: 'Yes ma'am, I did.' 'You washed nothing,' she says. And then I said: 'Ma'am, someday you'll be robbed or something like that and people say we [blacks, residents of *favelas*] just do that [use violence] but here you are cussing me out.' But she didn't want to hear any of that. She just got in her car and left. Just because I was black and from a *favela* . . . There are times when it makes you want to hate, but I just let it go . . . Like sometimes when I'm walking along Lagoa [the lake in the middle-class neighbourhood in Rio de Janeiro], some whites will like walk away from you when they come in my direction. Some will walk around a different way to avoid me . . . sometimes I'll talk to them. I'll say: 'Don't worry, I'm not a thief.' But they walk by looking at me like all strange.

I live just a few blocks from the church where João often watched and washed cars. Sometimes when walking or driving by I would say hello, but João was always slow to recognize me. He would see me first as a potential customer or a potential threat. Did I want a parking space? Might I be a middle-class person who was going to harass him? It took him a short time to register who I was, to put down the guard he had developed against possible harassment.

João relayed other frustrations, including losing the chance to play football for a junior league team associated with a professional team because he had no birth certificate. Whether he would have made it beyond the youth league teams to be a professional player is another question, but he had the talent to catch the eye of a recruiter of one of the major football teams.

João defined himself as different from other men in the community by his willingness to do whatever kind of work is required to keep his family fed, including shining shoes, parking cars and other odd jobs that some young men try to avoid or see as undignified, or beneath them. João also clearly identified the barriers he faces, including those that are specific to being a young, black man from a *favela*:

GB: How hard is it as a young man trying to find work?

JOÃO: It's harder for a man than a woman to find work, because . . . there are more opportunities for women, like an opening for being a cook . . . or someone to work a counter. They say they want a woman. A man will try, but there will be like this mistrust. 'Shit, he must be a thief.' Or like the boss will be racist and he doesn't want to let you [a black guy] work . . . it's easier for women. If they have an ID [identity card] they can get a job really fast.

Like the majority of young men in this setting, he also faced the constant threat of physical violence from two distinct sources: the police and the drug traffickers. João relayed various incidents of having been harassed and unfairly accused by police. Coping with drug-related violence was also an ongoing challenge. While João was not a part of a drug-trafficking gang, he lived near the border of two rival gangs. When asked what he does when gunfights break out in the neighbourhood, João emphasized the safety of his daughter and girlfriend:

GB: What do you do when shooting starts?

JOÃO : . . . what I do first is go by there [where his daughter and girlfriend live] and make sure everybody is at home. And if everybody is inside, then I go to my house [where his grandmother lives] and I stay there until it calms down. And then when it stops, I don't leave to go far away, I stay close. My biggest worry [when the shooting starts] is with my girlfriend.

Finding an alternative version of manhood

In spite of his lack of work, his anger over harassment by the middle class and the police, and having family members and friends involved in gangs, João stayed out:

GB: With you having cousins and friends in the *comandos*, why do you think you didn't participate in the *comando*?

JOÃO: . . . when I was 6, my father and mother and brothers and sisters . . . would all smoke [marijuana] and snort [cocaine]. And I stayed away from that from the time when I was little . . . And I had an aunt who was part of the *comando* and she brought up my cousins telling them: 'Don't do this when you grow up.' But they ended up in the *comando* . . . As for me, I already thought about this, reflected about it, even when I was 8 or 9. When I was [that age], I told my grandmother: 'Granny, if I get to be 17 or 18 and I never snort [cocaine], you can expect everything from me because then I'll never do it.' So then I kept my promise. I made it to 19 without smoking a cigarette or marijuana and without snorting [cocaine], without having a gun in my belt . . . But at 19 years, I never snorted or smoked.

GB: Did they ever directly invite you to join [the gangs]?

JOÃO: Yeah, I have one cousin [on this side of the neighbourhood, controlled by the Third Command] and one cousin [in the *comando*] on the other side [controlled by a rival gang, called the Red Command] . . . but I just turn them down. That's not what I want. I want to work because the day I have my daughter [living in my house with me], I want her to have the best education she can have, what I didn't have. I don't want this [the *comando* and drug-related violence] for her.

When asked if there was someone he looked up to or who was his inspiration for the kind of man he is – i.e. not involved in gangs and devoted to his partner and child – he answered:

> I look to my uncle. He's an engineer, like carpenter, does almost everything. He's never out of work. At home, he has the function of doing everything. He's always taking care of things, accepting responsibilities and he always makes sure that nothing is lacking at home.

João's ideal of what it means to be a man combines instrumental skills necessary for providing for a family – 'he does almost everything' – with a dedication to the needs of his family. In some ways, João was also able to see through the gender matrix. He was able to perceive how young women showed a preference for gang-involved young men as being 'real men' and thus attractive as partners, and how his version of a hard-working, family man was often seen by young women as uncool. João would openly criticize young women for the fact that they liked the guys in the gangs, that is that women liked the 'bad guys'. In one group setting with young women from his community present, he said:

> You see lots of hard workers without a woman, but you never see a gangster without a woman . . . you tell me [saying this to young women in the room] . . . there are lots of hard workers out there without a woman, but gangsters, they have a lot, a lot of women.

The young women in the room agreed with this, some of them looking a little embarrassed but admitting that the 'bad guy' was usually more attractive than the 'nice guy'. In another setting, he repeated this:

GB: Why do women like guys in the *comando*?

JOÃO: Because they have the best clothes. [A girl says]: 'Huh, I'm gonna go out with a guy without money? He doesn't give me anything.' But a gangster can give a motorcycle or whatever she wants because a gangster never goes without money, never goes out without money. But if a girl goes out with a hard worker, you know how it is, he'll have a hard time finding a job and getting money. So girls prefer to go out with the gangster.

Thus, João was highly aware that he was different, and of his projection of a non-violent and more gender-equitable identity or way of being a man. He also was able to identify the pressure or social sanctions that he sometimes faced for being this kind of man (being thought of as 'uncool'):

There's this guy who's a friend of mine and he had a girlfriend and she got pregnant and he abandoned her when she was pregnant, and he never liked to work, and he doesn't do anything, just takes from his mother. So his girl-friend had the baby and he doesn't work at all. He doesn't give anything to the baby, nothing for the girl, doesn't want to work. My point of view is dif-ferent . . . I want to be there when they need me, accepting my responsibil-ities. Even if I were to separate from the mother of my daughter and have another wife, I'm not gonna forget about my daughter . . . She'll always be first. But lots of young guys, they don't think about working, just think about stealing, using drugs, smoking . . . But me, not me. I stay away from that, drugs and smoking and stuff. If they think I'm uncool, so, okay, I'll be uncool then.

To mitigate the effects of feeling uncool, João became part of a peer group that supported non-gang-involvement and supported his being an involved father. The group offered him a safe place to be the kind of man he was trying to be.

Understanding pathways to resistance and resilience in settings of social exclusion

João could put words to the inner struggle about the kind of man he sought to be: a responsible, hard-working, family man versus a less-than-responsible young man (perhaps with ties to drug-trafficking gangs or at least emulating them to some degree). In one moment, reflecting about his parents and their drug use, João said:

My father is one of those guys that you say . . . okay, if you use drugs it's because of your parents. For me it's not your parents. It's the young person's own head. A youth thinks for himself. They know what's good and what's bad. I make my own conclusions. Just because my father did this . . . my father [used drugs], my brothers and sisters did. My mother did. My uncle too did it. If it were because of that, I'd be the biggest gangster in the neighbourhood. And I'm not. All I want to do is work . . . just work.

It is relevant to ask: how much disadvantage would most individuals take before becoming angry, turning to violence or becoming part of an armed group? Why shouldn't João be violent? Is it fear of being arrested, or fear in general? Is it a true sense of connection with several important people in his life: his grandmother, his girlfriend, his daughter? Clearly these issues are part of the story. João described his grandmother as giving him special attention that his cousins did not have, attention which may have helped him stay out of gangs. An easy-going temperament probably helps. João also does not have a physical appearance that might invoke stereotyped fear of low-income (mostly black) young men on the part of teachers or adults he may encounter. He showed positive, generally pro-social coping abilities. No doubt all of these issues contributed to his life directions.

João also seemed to see beyond the gender matrix. He could read the intentions of young men involved in drug trafficking, and the appeal of the 'bad guys' to young women. He saw others in his family who saw drug trafficking as a way to income and status and he saw the consequences. He was keenly aware that he lacked status, power and income – and that the drug-trafficking gangs could provide those – but he weighed the negative consequences and stayed out. He had at least one person in his family, his grandmother, with whom he had a special relationship. She seems to have treated him differently than his brothers and sisters. She encouraged his active involvement in his daughter's life. João has limited formal educational attainment, but he showed a kind of critical or reflective thinking. He was able to in effect step outside of himself and see how his life events affected him and consider his options for where he wanted to go. He showed metacognitive skills – that is he was able to think about how he thought – when weighing his life options. And he found one supportive family member and a reasonably supportive peer group who helped along the way.

This chapter begins with this example of João precisely because he exemplifies many of the pressures and strains that young men in such settings face: racism and classism; police harassment; finding a supportive peer group; family stresses; educational challenges; finding employment; and pressures associated with forming a family and caring for a child (often unplanned, but not necessarily unwanted). A given developmental risk or vulnerability rarely comes on its own; the literature on human development confirms that vulnerabilities often come in bundles, one leading to another, for example, poverty leading to family break-up, or the migration of a family member, or substance use. But João's story offers insights on how some young men can resist gravitating to violent versions of manhood, how youth also construct their own meaning and interpretation from their objective realities. From the story of João, we will look now at his community.

A favela called Maré

João's case study cannot speak for all individuals, and one specific low-income community cannot speak for all the other realities of low-income communities in Brazil, the United States, the Caribbean or Nigeria. Nonetheless, it does provide a useful backdrop for understanding the dimensions of social exclusion that young men face.

João comes from a neighbourhood called Nova Holanda, a low-income neighbourhood within a larger community called 'Complexo de Maré' (or 'Tide complex'), called tide because it borders the bay (Guanabara Bay) on which Rio de Janeiro sits. In the 1990 census, Maré had a total population of 106,000, making it one of the largest low-income 'complexes' in the city. It represents a mixture of working-class families, along with lower-income families, some of whom subsist on public food supplements from governmental or charitable organizations. Educational attainment is relatively low; fewer than one per cent of adults have any university education, compared to 16.7 per cent of adults in Rio de Janeiro overall. Adult illiteracy was 22 per cent, far higher than the national average.

Nova Holanda was formed in 1962 when the city government began forcibly removing entire *favelas* from the southern, middle-class part of the city (Silva 1995). Most of the original residents of Nova Holanda were immigrants to Rio from the northeast part of Brazil and the majority are of African or mixed descent (a mixture of Portuguese, African and indigenous Indian). All of the young men included in this study described themselves as black or mixed race.[4]

João and his peers represent the first generation of children born and raised in Nova Holanda. For most of their parents' generation, adolescence per se did not exist. In the previous generation, low-income young people were expected to complete only about six years of formal education and then to begin working. João and his friends are the first generation to have an adolescence – a prolonged moratorium involving additional formal education and time spent in recreational as opposed to economically productive activities. In short, while families in Maré are poor, many – probably most – have enough income to allow them to keep their children in school rather than have to work at early ages.

In a walk through Nova Holanda, the visitor sees a residential neighbourhood with unfinished, red brick two-storey dwellings in townhouse style. The townhouses face each other across narrow internal streets (though which cars cannot pass), bordered on other sides by wider streets designed for automobile traffic. In these narrower streets, at any time of the day residents sit outside their houses and children are playing. The streets are generally littered and the houses have no backyards or other fenced-in areas.

Interspersed with housing areas are open spaces, some of which hold run-down playground equipment and that are now filled with abandoned cars. Toward the major highway nearby are grassy areas, where on any given day boys are likely to be flying kites, playing soccer or taking care of emaciated horses.

The neighbourhood has several schools, large, uniformly constructed three-storey facilities of unfinished concrete. These are called CIEPs (in Portuguese, Centro Integrado de Educação Primaria, or Integrated Centres for Primary Education), built in the 1980s and nicknamed 'Brizolões' after the populist governor who had them commissioned. The CIEPs were designed to be complete primary educational facilities, with recreational areas, libraries and public health services. A visit to some of these CIEPs reveals considerable variation as to whether they live up to their promise of being complete, educational facilities. Some are tidy (albeit simple and with limited infrastructures), have libraries equipped with computers and books, and have well-kept classrooms; others are run down.

Moving west from the residential areas is the commercial part of Maré with grocers, pharmacies, beauty salons, auto repair shops and several larger commercial facilities. Immediately bordering the neighbourhood to the south is a large grassy area with football fields. In late 1999, the city government began construction of an Olympic Village, a large sporting complex meant to provide recreational activities for young people, although the nearby presence of gang activity means that many young people do not feel safe using it.

Since the 1980s, Maré, like other *favelas* in Rio de Janeiro, has lived in the face of drug-trafficking gangs (*comandos*) who traffic in cocaine and marijuana and engage in armed conflict over territory. In 1999–2000 Nova Holanda was 'occupied' by *Comando Vermelho* (the Red Command), one of the two largest drug-trafficking gangs in Rio de Janeiro. *Comando Vermelho*'s chief rival is *Terceiro Comando* (the Third Command), which occupies the adjacent community. In various *favelas* in Rio, these two rival groups (and others) clash over territory. To control or occupy a *favela* means that they sell drugs (to residents and others from outside the community), use the neighbourhood as a place to hide from police, live in the neighbourhood, recruit people from the neighbourhood and provide some minimal social benefits to the community, such as funding the local *samba* school or weekend dances (*baile funk*).

Residents tend to view the *comandos* with a mixture of fear, dislike, respect and admiration. *Comando* members are nearly all from the community, and while most residents oppose the violence, they also side with 'their boys' when violence breaks out between a rival *comando* or with police. The young men we worked with in Maré, for example, while seeking to define themselves as non-*comando*, sometimes had positive impressions of the *comando*. The *comando* was seen as bringing order to the community in the absence of effective governmental services and authority. The young men perceived the *comandos* as providing a useful, extra-official justice system that intervened in cases of interpersonal conflicts or domestic violence. For example, one young man called on the *comandos* when his girlfriend's previous boyfriend was stalking her.

From 1999 to 2004, there was what residents called a war going on between the two *comandos*. If the local leader of the *comando* is killed or imprisoned, a rival *comando* will often take this opportunity to invade the community and attempt to occupy its territory. During this period, there were several attempts by *Terceiro Comando* to invade Nova Holanda. For João and his peer group, the *comando* rivalry was particularly salient because most of them lived in the area of the neighbourhood that most closely borders the rival neighbourhood.

The school which the young men attended offers testimony to this violence; interior and exterior school walls have dozens of bullet holes. In one incident in early 1999, heavy shooting across the *comando* boundary took place during school hours, leading students to throw themselves on the floor. The school was closed for several days. Some teachers asked to be transferred or took medical leave. As a result, the school district built a chain fence on the side of the school that faced the rival *comando*. At the school entrance closest to the rival *comando*, one or two police cars and police officers toting large automatic weapons were frequently stationed.

The ongoing violence caused the young men to miss school, caused activities to be cancelled, led them to lose sleep and in one incident meant that most of the young men had to seek refuge with relatives or friends living in other neighbourhoods. In some sessions, the young men arrived rubbing their eyes and had difficulty staying awake.

This violence between rival *comandos* is ubiquitous to the point that young people in *favelas* throughout the city refer to themselves as being from '*Lado A*' or '*Lado B*' (the A side or the B side, referring to themselves as *Lado A*, and the rival group as *Lado B*). This notion of *Lado A* and *Lado B* leads to a two-front or three-front war: between the rival *comandos*, and between the police and each *comando*. Police invasion of the neighbourhood is feared as much or more than violence from the rival *comando*. Police are described as being violent, disrespectful of civilians (something the young men had frequently experienced and something we witnessed) and seldom worry about who is and who is not part of the *comando*. They break down doors, shoot without identifying suspects and often kill bystanders.[5] The media typically portray all the victims as *bandidos*, rarely using the word 'suspect'.

In 2000, the head of the *comando* in Nova Holanda was arrested. The rival *comando* perceived this as an opportune moment to invade. One evening, armed members of the rival *comando* (*Terceiro Comando*) entered Nova Holanda and began attempting to force their way into the houses of young men in the community who they believed were part of the *comando*. In one of these incidents, members of the rival *comando* from the adjacent neighbourhood invaded in the early hours of the morning, attacking homes of some members of the ruling *comando*. When the rival *comando* members encountered resistance and feared they would be trapped by police or members of the *Comando Vermelho*, they took a family hostage. They told the police that if they were not allowed to leave, they would kill their hostages. More than 200 police entered the community, closing off all entrances to the neighbourhood. Police were able to negotiate the release of the family and arrested the rival gang members.

During the incident, residents of Nova Holanda stood at the edges of the area the police had cordoned off shouting that the rival traffickers should be lynched. After police left with the rival gang members in custody, residents from the adjacent neighbourhood (the home base of the arrested traffickers) began to form a barricade along the border with Nova Holanda. They set tyres on fire and some began to arm themselves with rocks and sticks as if they would invade Nova Holanda. Residents of Nova Holanda, nervous that they would be attacked, called the police, whom they generally distrust and dislike, to restore order.

In 2003, a large police station was constructed in the neighbourhood, surrounded by high, barbed-wired walls. Within the first week it opened, a grenade was thrown into the compound. To ensure their safety, the police have allegedly sided with one of the gangs. Community members report that police sometimes pick up low-level drug traffickers from rival gangs and threaten to turn them over to the gang they are allied with – which would most likely mean execution – unless they or their family pays them 100 Brazilian *reais* (about US$36).

In late 2003, two youth in Nova Holanda were decapitated by the rival gang. Their killers played football with their heads. Their families had to bury them without heads. When the family asked the police if they would try to find the heads, the police reportedly asked for 200 *reais* (about US$72) for each. Shortly after that incident, a stray bullet from a shoot-out between rival gangs in Maré struck a middle-class woman who was driving on the nearby highway. The incident was widely reported in the press. The same weekend, five young people from the community were killed in gang-related violence. But there was no mention of their deaths in the major newspapers.

This short description may give the impression that Maré, and other low-income neighbourhoods like it around the world, are places of despair, violence and chaos. All of these things exist, to be sure, but Maré and other low-income urban settings like this are also spaces of socialization, of cultural production (music and other arts), sports and the pleasure of mixing with or hanging out with other young people like themselves. In spite of the violence described, young men say they value the company and friendships they have, and the sense of belonging. For all the doomsayers and newspaper headlines, most young men in these settings stay out of violence. Some actively speak out against it and work to help other young men stay out.

Growing up poor

A few pages of reflection about the life of one young man and one community is, of course, not enough to understand the complexities of these realities – and the subjective experiences of young people who live this structural disadvantage. But these details give some sense of what social exclusion means in detailed terms and of how it wears on young people. And in Brazil, and other settings that will be described in this book, it wears on far too many.

With a population of more than 170 million, Brazil is the world's tenth largest economy, and has an economy characterized by extreme social divisions. According to World Bank (1997) figures, Brazil has the world's worst income distribution among more than 60 countries for which data are available. As of 1989, the richest 10 per cent of the population controlled 51.3 per cent of total income, while the poorest 20 per cent of the population had access to just 2.1 per cent of total income (World Bank 1997). Approximately one-third of the Brazilian population lives in a situation of absolute poverty, and about half of Brazil's young people (ages 18 and under) live in poverty (Ribeiro and Saboia 1994; Bercovich et al. 1998).

On some measures, life is improving for the poor in Brazil, but social exclusion continues to mean unmet needs for adequate housing, sanitation, education, health and other services. Growing to manhood in a place like this means, as will be shown in greater detail, too little schooling, too few jobs and too few options for achieving a respected, socially recognized masculine identity apart from gang involvement. For girls, early childbearing is commonplace, not because of lack of contraceptives or health services, but mostly for the lack of something else or some other role that gives them status and meaning in life.

Few young people in these settings are able to climb socially, or acquire university education. Brazilian researcher and former Maré resident Jailson de Souza e Silva (2003) examined the life stories of several individuals from Maré who were able to attend university and acquire stable, government-employed jobs. The common factors involved in achieving this educational attainment were staying removed or away from the street culture, generally some family support (often differentiated for each child in the family), finding allies or supportive teachers and learning how the educational system worked. Their life stories tell of overcoming tremendous odds, of facing racial and class discrimination and of setbacks and frustrations; most of the individuals required more than the usual four or five years to finish a university education.

Young people interviewed in these settings are keenly aware of the odds against them. For some young men, becoming a gang member provides a sense of belonging, a source of income and status by being feared. Frustration over social exclusion and fear – of police, of the middle class – are turned on their heads. Young men in gangs seem to say: 'Instead of me fearing you, you'll fear me.' Gang members achieve status through force and brutality, but they achieve status.

As mentioned at the beginning of this chapter, young people are also keenly aware of the false or exaggerated promises of capitalist democracies. Since the early 1990s, Brazil has seen the advent of mobile phones, cable TV, triple the number of brands of cars and other imported and nationally produced goods. Billboards with these goods line the major avenue that borders Maré. The once heavily protected market and economy of Brazil has opened up to globalization, as happened in India and many other developing countries. Aggressive trade practices from the United States and Western Europe and development policies supported by the International Monetary Fund and World Bank have opened the doors of an unprecedented range of goods and advertising of those goods. There are new jobs and new industries – for some. For too many, like João, these promises of goods to make their lives better, to attract girls and to be real men, remain well out of reach.

Chapter 4

The trouble with young men

Coming of age in social exclusion

The realities of poverty described in the previous chapter are, unfortunately, strikingly similar in many other low-income, urban areas around the world. Poverty and its effects vary tremendously by country and setting, and it is impossible to adequately sum up the socioeconomic realities of diverse parts of the world in a few paragraphs. However, social exclusion plays out in similar ways in the Caribbean, parts of Africa and in low-income settings in the United States.

Limin' in the Caribbean

In the Caribbean, for example, roots of young men's sense of exclusion can be found in the economic difficulties of the region since the early 1980s. While the details vary by island, the small economies of virtually every country in the region suffered during the 1980s and 1990s. Many of the islands subsisted on one or two main export goods – bananas, bauxite, sugar cane – all of which were subjected to major price swings. Along with international market forces, structural adjustment policies led to a decline in government spending for social services, including education and health services – factors which had a direct impact on low-income youth. Women have fared slightly better in the service industry, including the tourism trade (which also suffers from market forces), and hence show higher rates of employment than young men, as well as higher rates of educational attainment. Among the results of these trends is internal and international migration, which places tremendous stress on families. One young man from Jamaica, who subsisted on short-term jobs, had the following to say about the situation:

> There are lots of places that want to pay you nothing [for working]. They use and abuse you . . . some fire you overnight. You don't have a future, because they don't care about you. Everybody is working for today, because you don't know about tomorrow.
>
> (Geoff, 17, African Caribbean, Kingston, Jamaica)

While statistics serve to document economic and social trends in the region, certain qualitative factors must be emphasized to fully understand the situation of young men in the Caribbean. Among young men interviewed, the mood was one of disillusionment and a lack of hope. The failures of the 'system' – both economic and political – have left many Caribbean young men with little hope for the future and little belief in the ability of a given youth programme, organization or initiative to make a difference in their lives.

Young men throughout the Caribbean can be seen 'limin'', hanging out on the streets, at the beach, in parks or in rum bars, with nothing to do and no place to go. They are keenly aware of political corruption and the lack of educational and employment opportunities in the region. They also perceive that those who made a living illicitly, drug traffickers and producers, go unpunished (and that some political leaders in the region collude with them). The attitudes and postures of these youth also reflect the influence of media images from Europe and North America and a perceived pressure to keep up with the latest trends – a consumer-oriented version of what it means to be a man. As an out-of-school young man from Trinidad and Tobago said:

> I'm sceptical, you know, that things will change. If we see youth in the U.S.A. doing it, we think we have to do it. You know they call Trinidad 'Little America'? . . . So if we see it on TV in the U.S.A. we have to do it here, like youth carrying guns to school so we have to carry guns to school. So, if you can't help youth there [in the United States], how are they going to help youth here? You can't even stop the drug pushers.
>
> (Peter, 18, African Caribbean, Port of Spain, Trinidad)

Trying to make it in the 'hoods and the barrios in the United States

In the United States, the social exclusion of young men in the school setting and workplace, particularly for low-income African American young men, has been widely documented in other studies. Researcher Ann Arnett Ferguson (2000) in her interviews and interactions with African American boys in public schools describes in detail the unequal punishment meted out against them, and the challenge of boys succeeding in school when such achievement was seen as 'selling out' or 'playing white'.

North American sociologists Elijah Anderson (1990) and William Julius Wilson (1996) have highlighted how the loss of blue collar jobs in factories and industrial work settings led to a rapid decline in social capital and a shortage of gainfully employed black men to serve as role models for young men. The 'old heads' – older men who could show younger men the way to adult manhood – lost their status. Men moved for work or abandoned families when they felt they could not provide for them (or felt compelled to leave so that mothers could receive public aid, conditioned for many years in the United States on the absence of a man in the household). One result was that gangs grew in strength, filling a void in social capital, socialization and status for many young men.

In Chicago, interviews were carried out in precisely these kind of neighbourhoods, with young men from three different low-income neighbourhoods, all either African American or Latino (both Puerto Rican and Mexican) young men.[1] The low-income African American neighbourhood in Chicago where young men were interviewed is characterized by female-headed households, a reliance on the extended kinship network, high unemployment and early childbearing (teenage childbearing), which is generally not accompanied by the formation of a stable union. As of the early 1990s, the low-income African American community where the high school is located had an unemployment rate of 34.1 per cent compared to 11.6 per cent for the city as a whole. Nearly two-thirds of the population was classified as living in poverty, compared to about one-fifth of Chicago as a whole. In one public housing setting in the community, an estimated eight out of ten households were headed by women. In this situation of resource scarcity, relationships between men and women are sometimes strained, and domestic violence, primarily by men against women – but also in some cases by women against men – was reported to be common. In Chapters 8 and 9, tensions in male–female relationships in low-income settings will be discussed in greater detail.

Various researchers have provided insights, both in the United States and to a lesser extent in the United Kingdom, on how a lack of employment, accompanied with systematic discrimination, contributes to some low-income African American (in the case of the United Kingdom, African and Caribbean) men's abandonment of their families, and their adoption of what some authors have called a 'cool pose' version of masculinity. This is an exaggerated masculine version of self that serves as a coping mechanism to maintain 'face' or self-respect in the face of racism – particularly forms of racism that specifically demasculate black men – and in the absence of other sources of male identity and self-worth (Majors and Billson 1993). In sum, truncated employment possibilities, plus historical racism and social exclusion, are related to some of the violent, versions of masculinities found in such settings.

The Hispanic community where young men were interviewed represents a slightly different scenario. In many cases, men migrated (from Mexico or Central America) first for work, and sent remittances back to their families. As the men established themselves (sometimes with legal status, sometimes not), they often brought their families to the United States as well. Many of these families replicate some of the gendered patterns found in Mexico in terms of traditional divisions of household labour and rigid male and female roles. Generational conflicts are reported to be common as fathers in particular raise daughters in a setting where women are granted far more freedom than in rural parts of Mexico and Central America.

As in the case of the African American community, early childbearing is common, but is generally accompanied by a common law union. Unemployment is similarly high but there is a greater tendency of recent immigrants to accept minimum wages jobs and a prevailing discourse that the opportunities available – however limited – are still better than conditions in rural Mexico and Central America.

Some Hispanic fathers faced a different kind of 'loss of face' than the African American men. Specifically, they found that their roles as heads of households were limited by a public education and social service system that regulated certain practices – particularly the use of physical violence against children or women – and in effect, reduced their traditional paternal power. Nonetheless, men were in general more visibly present in Hispanic households than the African American ones.

'They think we are hooligans': Young men and social exclusion in Nigeria

Communities in sub-Saharan Africa (with a few exceptions such as Botswana) are generally much poorer than the other three areas presented here and in some ways difficult to compare to settings in North America, the Caribbean and South America. In Nigeria, which is wealthier than some of its neighbors because of oil revenue, access to public education and public health services is much lower (than in Latin America, North America and the Caribbean), while unemployment and underemployment is much higher than in Latin America and the Caribbean. Nigeria also has a history of regional conflicts that intertwine with religious conflicts (Muslims in the north of the country versus Christians and indigenous religions in the southern part of the country), and young men often find themselves drawn into and participating in this violence. Most young men are also keenly aware of the widescale corruption in Nigeria, particularly the squandering of oil revenues, and highlight the loss of trust in leadership and ability of government to make a real difference in their lives.

In this setting, most young people and adults said that 'schemes' were required to acquire jobs, which generally meant knowing someone in the public sector or paying a bribe. Some low-income men told of having paid such bribes to get jobs, particularly to get one of the highly coveted public service jobs. Young men also said that for women, acquiring employment and career advancement in general means accepting sexual harassment and exchanging sexual favours. One young man said:

> Even school boys and university boys have to rob. There are those boys at that university [mentioned name] who have guns on them, because they

need to rob just to be able to pay their school fees. Young people need an income. [But we know] that the leaders do not want young people to move ahead. They want them to be dependent.

(Halim, out-of-school, young man, age 20, Kaduna, Nigeria)

Young men also related their involvement in the ethnic and religious violence that has been prevalent in contemporary Nigeria. Young men in the city of Kaduna – which lies along the tension line between Muslim and Christian groups – told stories of their involvement in such violence. Many were instigated into joining by being told that 'Muslims are killing our Christian brothers' and vice versa. Some young men were bussed in by different religious groups and paid – in the form of food – to participate in riots and protests. Many of the young men could clearly associate their involvement in this violence with the fact that they had nothing else to do and nothing to lose if they participated. One low-income Muslim man in his late thirties who had only recently acquired a low-level civil servant job, and was content with that, said:

Since 1981 I have been involved in every riot there has been. If the violence [between Christian and Muslim youth] came, I would be involved. I had no work. I had nothing to do. Why should I not get involved? Three months ago, I became employed as a civil servant. Now that I am getting my daily bread, why should I get involved [in such violence]? Lots of young men do not have this [stable work].

(Mohammed, civil servant, age 38, Kaduna, Nigeria)

Similarly, a young male secondary school student, talking about why young men get involved in this ethnic-related violence, said:

It is education and illiteracy. If you find those who take part in the violence, you will see they are illiterate. If you give them a little money to be involved for him to get involved, they will get involved. But if you think about being a doctor [that is becoming a doctor in the future] tomorrow, I don't think you are going to want to get involved in this because you know you might die.

(Franklin, age 17, secondary school student, Kaduna, Nigeria)

International data suggest that as many as 70 million young people aged 15–24 are currently unemployed, and that between 2004 and 2014, 500 million young people will enter the world's workforce. While rates vary by country, by urban–rural settings and by educational attainment, among other variables, limited data suggest that youth employment is two to three times higher than adult unemployment, worldwide and in Africa (Okojie 2003).

As a result of this unemployment and underemployment, many young men in Nigeria describe being in a kind of limbo: unable to marry because they did not have a stable income and unable to find stable employment. They take unpaid apprenticeships, carry out odd jobs, and struggle to find spaces in schools – if they are fortunate, in university. However, even university youth, who generally came from families with slightly more income, complain that a university education did not guarantee employment.

In addition to employment struggles, young men in Muslim–Christian conflict areas say that they try to stay away from the sectarian violence that periodically flares up. Their average day is filled with tremendous idle time, hanging out with not much to do and limited prospects for the next day:

ALFRED: When I left school, I was an apprentice [unpaid], and I learned a little about working. I was not idle. I found work fast, but it is very difficult and offers meagre pay.

MOHAMMED: My father was a painter and I used to go with him on his work. When he died, I followed my father's friends [also painters] on some odd jobs. But I have had no job since 2000 [this was 2003]. When I'm not working, I do small work, bricklaying, building, digging. Sometimes I have work, other times not.

ALI: If I have no work, I try to spend my time reading, bettering myself, reading in Hausa and English.

AYO: I do odd jobs. At times, if I don't have work, I go with my brother who is a welder. And when I have no work, I watch films.

JOSEPH: Sometimes I work. When I don't have work, I play football. The bad part is, sometimes the police harass us. [*Why?*] Because we have no work and they think we are hooligans.

To be sure, the realities of the four areas studied are far more complex than presented here. Nonetheless, these examples give a general sense of the nature of social exclusion, and the specific realities of low-income, urban-based young men in these settings. Community violence is a constant in all four communities, as are clashes with law enforcement.

Young men in these settings joke around, hang out with their friends, find girlfriends, listen to music, watch television, play football or other sports and participate in religious organizations; indeed, these are the things they say give their lives meaning. But they also demonstrate high degrees of anger, disillusionment and modest to little hope for the future.

Direct encounters with racism and classism

As mentioned in Chapter 3, living in situations of poverty and unemployment and underemployment is not simply a problem of material deprivation. Class divisions limit the movement of young people and can leave them with a hypervigilant attitude when travelling from their low-income neighbourhoods to middle-class parts of the city, which is nearly always seen as risky – in all of these settings. Young men from socially marginal neighbourhoods recount numerous examples of having encountered harassment from police or some degree of classism. In the United States and Brazil, harassment and classism is also tied closely to racism. Young men described having been the victims of shame and gave a clear sense that challenging racism or classism in any way would make things even worse.

In the case of Maré, for example, many of the young men and their parents rightly feared that ventures outside the *favela* entailed risking hostility, violence or discrimination. Some of the young men frequently went outside the community because of work. Some went to the beaches in the southern part of the city or to Maracanã stadium to see football matches – both of which are among the few spaces in Rio de Janeiro where individuals of all social classes mix. These excursions outside of the *favela* led to encounters with racist and classist individuals. On one field trip to use a recreational facility, a woman called one of the boys a *favelado*, a term that while literally correct and on its surface inoffensive (it literally means someone from a *favela*), has derogatory connotations meaning that the individual is uneducated, of lower-class status and potentially criminal. The young man concerned, aged 13, replied: 'And you wonder why people from *favelas* rob people like you?'

On one occasion, the young men were invited to a presentation at the Municipal Theatre in downtown Rio de Janeiro, generally a place that only middle- and upper-middle-class individuals frequent. When they entered the theatre, a white, middle-class adult looked at one of the young men in the group and said: 'I didn't know *favelados* came to things like this.' The young man (Ronaldo) said that he simply engaged in eye contact with the person, but said nothing. On another occasion, Ronaldo reported being present at a robbery at a bus stop. When word circulated around the bus stop, arriving passengers assumed that Ronaldo and his friend – being African Brazilian – were responsible.

When the young men travel by public bus together, they disperse to several parts of the bus. Passengers around them observed this group of young, black (and low-income) men getting on the bus and looked tense. When asked why they disperse like this on the bus, the young men said that they do not scare the other passengers as much when they sit apart. At the same time, if someone tries to get on the bus to rob, they can look out for each other – not with the intention of using violence against would-be assailants but so they can leave the bus as soon as possible.

Confrontations with racist individuals and prejudiced remarks lead these young men to seek comfort in numbers when they travel outside the community, and explains why some of them prefer to stay in their communities. The young men appreciated the outings offered as part of our activities with them, because our presence as middle-class professionals offered them some protection from these racist and classist comments and from police harassment.

When going outside the community, the young men also tend to dress differently; rather than wearing their usual outfit of baggy shorts, a sleeveless T-shirt and sandals, they often wear long trousers or dressier Bermuda shorts. They told us that they sought to demonstrate that they were not boys from the *favela*, or not the stereotypical version of boys from the *favela* in any case, and thus not to be feared and had the right to circulate in these other spaces. One young man – a university student from a low-income neighbourhood in one of the satellite cities that rings Brasilia – said:

> People don't know what it's like growing up in the neighbourhoods where we come from. In one of the schools we work in there is drug trafficking and girls who have to sell sex . . . Youth here have low esteem. They walk hunched over. Their skin looks bad and damaged because of malnutrition and exposure to the sun. We don't have the clothes that make us look [middle class] . . . We change the way we dress when we go into town [to be more formal] . . .
>
> I'll give you an example. One time when we went to town to this restaurant, they thought we were parking boys [boys who park cars]. A friend of mine who used to work as a parking boy said that when he worked parking cars at McDonald's, middle-class boys would come back to their cars and throw French fries on the ground to them . . . Can you imagine that? Treating them like they were pigeons or something.
>
> (Marcelo, university student, African Brazilian, Brasilia, Brazil)

Perhaps the most insidious side of the discrimination the young men faced was that which took place in their own community. Within Maré, for example, young men sometimes encountered prejudiced attitudes for the fact of being young men and thus having a presumed connection to *comandos*. In general, there were few social institutions in the community where a group of young men – sometimes noisy, sometimes unruly, but rarely threatening nor violent – was truly welcomed. Staff at the health clinics were observed turning the young men away because they were not wearing shirts. I witnessed disparaging and frightened looks of teachers when they entered the school as a group. Indeed, the only social institution in the community that seemed to truly welcome them were the evangelical churches. At one point, nearly all the young men who participated in the group activities we organized were attending one of the evangelical churches. Only two of the young men seemed to be truly 'converted'; the rest said they went mainly as a social activity. It was something to do in one of the few, non-violent spaces in the community that invited them.

What is the impact of this discrimination and exclusion? Some of the young men showed anger in their voices when talking about individuals from middle-class backgrounds. In the case of Brazil, the young men occasionally said negative things about 'playboys', the term they used for young men their age from middle-class backgrounds. But in general their discourses and affect did not suggest the level of anger seen in young African American men in Chicago. Young men and African American teachers and staff on the South Side of Chicago were at times openly hostile toward the white middle class. There was a palpable discourse of having been denied something – the middle-class North American dream – and white middle-class North America was to blame. Young men in the garrison communities of Kingston, Jamaica, often showed a similar anger toward the African Caribbean middle class and toward white tourists. The anger in their looks and comments is meant to be perceived and to intimidate. In Nigeria, young men showed a disdain for older men, particularly those they called the 'elite' and the *Al-hajis*, a term referring to Muslim men who had made the pilgrimage to Mecca (an indication that they have some wealth). This frustration has probably increased as the physical trappings of the globalized middle class have become more visible and more available for some.

Some of the young men in all of these settings, however, described their encounters with classism, racism and prejudice as being a nuisance, but these events did not apparently leave them with a sense of anger toward the world around them. In many cases, the young men seemed to find peer groups who shared a similar way of coping. They sought and found optimistic peers, teachers or other adults who presented them with discourses of hope, perseverance and solidarity.

Your friendly neighbourhood law enforcement system

Young men in Rio de Janeiro, Chicago, Kingston (and elsewhere in the English-speaking Caribbean) and Kaduna all had highly formed and overwhelmingly negative views toward police and law enforcement. They were aware of the ways in which this system unfairly and unequally treats them, compared to their middle-class counterparts. Many of them – if they did not have personal experience – had also seen brothers, cousins and friends unjustly treated and mistreated through false arrests to brutality.

An example from the Caribbean illustrates this. St Vincent and Grenadines has a population of about 100,000 and survives mostly by selling bananas (which bring a fairly low value on the world market). A few small villages live by whaling and fishing. It feels in many ways like one large Caribbean village, where everyone knows everyone and informal social control still works. When a drunken man asked me for money, an 'auntie' (older woman) immediately chastised him and swung her handbag at him. Like most of the Caribbean, there are many idle young men, most of whom have dropped out of school earlier than their sisters and female peers. Many young men are lured into substance use and drug selling.

These same young men were keenly aware of the two social institutions filled with other young men who had been caught selling or using drugs. One was the overcrowded prison (in the late 1990s, there was only one for this island country of about 100,000 residents), where the arms and faces of the young black men could be seen just beyond the shadows of the barred windows. These same windows looked onto the crystalline shoreline just a short distance away and onto the port area where cruise ships arrive daily. This was not a prison hidden away in some country town, but instead was a visible, centrally located reminder to young men of what would happen if they strayed.

The other place for wayward young men in St Vincent was the mental hospital, where nurses administered psychotropic medication to mostly young men, even when their only 'mental illness' was having been caught using marijuana. Young men commented that the 'bigshots' could always buy their way out of jail; they were aware of the collusion of high-level government officials in drug smuggling. They were highly aware that the criminal justice system was for those who could not buy their way out.

In Chicago, young men knew about new and tougher laws for drug-related crimes that were enacted in the United States in the 1980s and 1990s; they could frequently cite the statistic that a black man was more likely to end up in jail in the United States than to go to university. Sometimes the justice system was subtle in its warnings; at other times it openly took its threat directly to young people.

At a seminar for students from several schools from mostly African American neighbourhoods organized by the prosecutor's office, there were presentations by African American men who were victims of gun-related violence and who gave testimonials to young people about staying out of violence. Most of the men were paralysed from the waist down and wheelchair-bound. Some had been involved in criminal activity; others were simply in the wrong place at the wrong time. One had a colostomy as a result of his gunshot and described what that was like. Throughout the seminar, participants fidgeted in their seats. Then a white prosecutor came to the podium and showed pictures of dead black men and enjoined youth not to get involved in these kind of activities, because, he said: 'Sooner or later we find you . . .'

The spectacle of several black men in wheelchairs and the slides of dead men were useful attention-getters, for about 10 minutes. Mostly, the message was taken as more of the same. The young people were counting the minutes until the seminar ended. Those who did not have watches asked me for the time, or looked round at a clock on the back wall. Conversations focused on: When is the break? When does the bus come? The adults who organized the event seemed to think this would be a life-altering experience for the audience. They were seemingly unaware that these African American youth had heard this all before. The young people knew that bullets maimed and killed and that black men are the mostly likely victims and perpetrators of this violence. Indeed, they had heard the warning so many times that it ceased to have much meaning.

In Kaduna, Nigeria, there was also a clear perception that the justice system was skewed in favour of the middle class. Police were seen as repressive and violent, often causing violence from rioting or clashes between rival ethnic groups or rival religious groups to get even worse. Violent police and soldiers were seldom punished for excessive use of force. During a visit to Kaduna, the UN had arranged a police escort for myself and a colleague. We asked the police escort to sit outside or stay away during our discussions with the young men; a policeman carrying a rifle does not tend to leave youth at ease to talk. In one session, the police officer simply walked into a group discussion. I suggested that the young people might be more comfortable if he waited outside, but one said, causing laughter in the group: 'We are Nigerian youth. The police don't scare us. We're used to them.'

Young men in all four settings recounted incidents of maltreatment by the police. One African American young man in Chicago said this:

GB: Have you ever had a run in with the police?

TAMIR: Yes, it happened at the end of this hallway. A police beat me up. He was the head of the CAP [the Community Area Policing programme, the branch of the police that was supposed to establish positive relations with the community]. He told me that I was being disrespectful to the assistant principal. And he took me around the corner [and] punch [sic] me in stomach and choke me telling me 'little nigger, I will kill you' and when I told him I am going to call the police he said: 'I am the police.' And this is not the first run in with the police. I come to my grandmother [sic] house on 53rd and State and the gangbangers was running from the police because they selling drugs so they [the police] ask me questions saying I look like I was affiliated with the gangs.

Such stories were also common in Brazil, where police were described as being as brutal as, and more corrupt than, *comando* members. One young man, who had been involved in drug trafficking, said he was taken to an abandoned house where police tortured him to force him to identify accomplices, and then asked him for money:

GINALDO: [Once when I was selling drugs] they [the police] took me off in this corner, said lots of things, took me to this house that was under construction. Then they took me to the police station, violated me.

GB: You mean the police?

GINALDO: Yeah. They terrorized me. They wanted money. So I went to try to get some money so they would let me go.

A young man in Brazil relayed this event:

> I was arrested . . . they handcuffed me in the cell . . . I was hungry . . . didn't give me anything to eat . . . when I left the next morning I was starving. They didn't give me water or anything. Didn't explain anything to me . . . they said they picked me up because I was trying to take money from this old man. The man was giving me money . . . then another time, I was getting on a bus, this cop put a gun to my head for no reason.
>
> (Alex, 19, African Brazilian, Rio de Janeiro, Brazil)

Another young man in Brazil described being picked up by police, who mistook him for someone else who was robbing the bus:

> I felt ashamed [when the police were searching us] because there were all these people waiting at the bus stop . . . and I was being held like with my arms behind my back like I was a thief, but I wasn't. So then they searched my pockets and asked who . . . was with me . . . and asked if we were robbing the bus and we said no. And then they said that if they ever caught us committing a crime they were gonna kill us, that they would tear our heads off.
>
> (Bruno, 17, African Brazilian, Rio de Janeiro, Brazil)

In one neighbourhood in Rio de Janeiro, where we spoke with young men, 29 per cent of nearly 450 men aged 15–60 interviewed said they had been arrested or picked up by police at least once. It is hard to imagine that nearly one-third of men in the community had been involved in criminal activity. To be sure, some of the young men admitted to being involved in antisocial activities occasionally, but even in those incidents, the police response was exaggerated to the point of brutality. One young man said he was apprehended by police for painting graffiti on a bridge near Rio's international airport:

> They [the police who picked us up] started to hit us . . . one said he was going to set us on fire . . . so they put alcohol on all our feet and then he lit a match and threw it down and we all jumped up and stamped our feet and kept the fire from getting on us . . . then they took us to the police station . . . yelling at us all the time.
>
> (Pedro, 15, African Brazilian, Rio de Janeiro, Brazil)

In sum, for many young men in all of these settings, the police and law enforcement system were seen as a threat as big or bigger than other forms of violence around them, and seen as representing an indifferent middle class, or in the case of Nigeria and the Caribbean, serving the interests of corrupt politicians. In group settings, young men sometimes swapped these stories about their encounters with police, often starting with a 'one time' or 'me too'. There was a sense of normalcy that this is how police are. To be harassed or picked up at least once – and to live to tell about it – was just another rite of passage on the way to manhood.

'There are no men in my family apart from me'

Material want or poverty is rarely the only challenge that low-income families face; poverty often fragilizes families and brings with it numerous other vulnerabilities. In Chicago, as previously noted, in one of the neighbourhoods, four out of five families were headed by women. Among one group of twenty-four young men I worked with in Brazil, seven did not know their fathers; half lived in single-mother households. These are crude indicators of family vulnerability to be sure; at times having a man, particularly if he was violent, was worse than not having a man and the income he may have represented. The following are some typical descriptions of the young men about their family circumstances, suggesting instability, health problems and early death (exacerbated in situations of poverty):

> When I was 9 my mother and father started having marital problems. My father started hitting her . . . I was living in Mexico then but then I went to live with my grandmother. That was a good moment [living with my grandmother]. When I was 10, I came to live with my father [who had since moved to Chicago].
>
> (Armando, 19, Hispanic, Chicago)

> My momma was like my backbone. I played football or basketball and she was always there. She was there for everything I did. My dad was not. So when she died [of carbon monoxide poisoning], they had this funeral and everybody thought I was gonna be like I was gonna snap. All I could do is sit there and look at my momma.
>
> (Reed, 19, African American, Chicago)

> My mother abandoned me when I was like 3 months old . . . But I had a mother figure growing up. At like 12 or 13, I was homeless. I was living in a friend's van. I was like house hoppin', you know. And then I went to live with a real close friend's family . . . so they're like my family.
>
> (Kique, 22, Hispanic, Chicago)

A young man in Brazil told the story of men in his family, all of which read like a case study on men's health and mortality in low-income neighbourhoods. His father was murdered, and two of his stepfathers died from alcohol abuse. Matter-of-factly, he concluded: 'There are no men in my family apart from me.' The figures of men's higher mortality rates seem distant, and even low when seen on a table of figures. But for many families these health risks are lived and breathed.

Most young men in the United States, Brazil and the Caribbean told of someone in the family who held things together in vulnerable moments or crisis situations, such as the death of a parent, family violence, a substance use problem by a parent, or loss of a job. Typically, this person who held things together was a grandmother, an aunt or a mother, but occasionally also a father, stepfather or uncle. Notably, there were rarely two or three persons reported as being the backup systems for the family. In the majority of cases, when stress came, which was commonplace in settings of social exclusion, the task of holding a family together and providing adequate income, care and protection fell on just one person. This dependency on one person leads to situations of tremendous vulnerability. Many young men in all four settings described life-altering events when this individual died, or became incapacitated in some way. These events – death of a mother or grandmother, or death or incarceration of a father – were sometimes described as being the trigger points for young men becoming involved in gang-related violence.

Gotta have those Nikes

For most young men in these settings, families struggle to provide food, clothing and shelter. As if that were not enough, young people – including those in low-income neighbourhoods – are the deliberate targets of marketers. This primarily includes brands of clothing targeted specifically for low-income youth, and the ubiquitous Nike shoes. Young men experience stress over not having the 'right' brand of shoes. Among young men in Brazil, in outings, they would worry whether they looked nice or had the right shoes or clothes. They would spend an entire month's income on one shirt with a Nike or similar logo on it, and take out credit to buy Nike shoes. When Nike introduced a new football shoe (costing about 500 Brazilian *reais*, or about US$180), sales representatives showed the shoe at football fields where young men from *favelas* play. There was no apparent contradiction in their minds, nor of the young men interested in the shoes, that the cost of the shoes was what their parents earned in a month.

Young men rarely commented openly about this marketing that targeted them; it seemed as natural to them as being young. Even the poorest, out-of-school young men in low-income Muslim neighbourhoods in Nigeria were wearing Chicago Bulls T-shirts with the National Basketball Association logo (probably counterfeit). In being at the economic margins of society, it was central to these young men to be able to signify that they were part of the consumer society. You could wear the same brand as the middle class – even if you had only one Nike T-shirt and had to wash it every two days to use it, or even if you took your Nikes off as soon as you returned home so you did not wear them out.

For better or worse, international mass marketing has made Nikes and other similar brands part of an international youth culture that crosses class and country boundaries. There may be some democracy to be found in this situation: if you can buy at least one T-shirt or pair of shoes with the right brand, you can be part of something – a globalized youth culture – no matter how poor you may be. However, it is clear that young men experienced pressure and stress when they were not able to be a part of this international, consumer-oriented youth culture. Sometimes, they could not buy Nikes; sometimes, they said, they had to sell their Nikes to buy cooking gas. Sometimes, their one brand-name shirt was dirty and they felt inadequate to leave their neighbourhood.

Young people in most of the world experience some pressure to fit in, to buy the same brands and dress the same as their peers. Increasingly this pressure is globalized; even low-income youth want to fit in. For young people who lack the income to buy the right brands, this pressure can be a source of stress and frustration.

Coping in the face of social exclusion

With these somewhat common backdrops, how do young men cope with this social exclusion? Some young men vent their frustration through violence, or gravitate toward a peer group that encourages violence. Most of the young men, however, find at least some positive, or pro-social ways for coping.

Interviews with young men in Brazil and the United States suggest that some young men had found positive outlets for discussing personal problems and concerns. Some of the African American young men interviewed in Chicago and Rio de Janeiro found spaces in group activities or via cultural expression. Several of the young men in this group were involved in rap, hip hop, *pagode* and other forms of music; for these young men rap and other musical forms was an important (and apparently positive) outlet for expression and for venting frustrations and problems that emerged from their personal lives. This highlights the important role of culture (or its potential role) – and in this case the specific African cultural tradition of oral history and music – in helping make sense of frustration, pain and challenges faced.

African American young men in Chicago said they could talk to a family member, a friend or someone at school (a teacher or counsellor) when they felt the need to talk. Some Hispanic young men in Chicago found it more difficult to talk about these personal losses and stresses and had fewer spaces where they could talk about them. For most of the young men in Chicago, early family losses or separations continued to be a source of pain. Furthermore, many of the young men were able to make a mental connection between that loss or stress in the past and their current drive and actions. In several cases, the young men could articulate the strategies they used in the past and those they currently use to deal with personal stress. This ability to reflect about their survival strategies and to connect their past loss to the present may seem to be an obvious point, but many young men cannot articulate or reflect about these strategies or do not have them.

In the case of young men in Brazil, there was a tremendous importance in being able to state publicly in a group of male peers that they had experienced pain and fear. In various group discussions, when we simply asked young men to talk about violence they had witnessed, the session could easily last up to two hours as young men traded stories of violence they had lived, witnessed or heard about it. Many of these sessions seemed to be cathartic in the sense of being able to swap stories and comfort each other in having lived to tell the tale.

The peer group was key to coping with social exclusion in all four settings. In Maré, the young men we worked with formed a non-gang gang, that is a gang that was not involved in drug trafficking. Their peer group or clique reinforced a mostly non-violent and non-*comando* identity. For a time, some of the young men called themselves United in Peace (after a rap song they composed against community violence). One young man said this about the group:

GB: What do you like about the group [your peer group]?
JEFERSON: . . . We're all friends and we don't act like clowns [and] fight with each other. We're always together, always ready to help the other. We never get upset with the other. Sometimes there will be a fight, but not like a fight to break up a friendship . . . We [this group] never do anything really wrong. The only thing we do is play around sometimes, you know like adolescents, shouting and stuff. We always try to value what's good in our community, trying to do our best for people around here in Nova Holanda.

In addition to reinforcing a non-violent group identity, this specific peer group showed affection (as much as adolescent boys do) and support for each other. Some of the older members seemed to protect the younger members. Several of the young men described incidents in which they had helped each other in difficult moments. One young man described being comforted by the group when he had been arguing with his mother, and said that he was able to cry in front of another member of the group. Another young man had witnessed severe violence by his stepfather against his mother and was able to confide in members of the group.

Most of the young men seemed to appreciate the sense of protection that this peer group offered. For many young people in *favelas*, forming a *bonde* or a gang – violent, non-violent or somewhere in between – can be an effective way to protect oneself both within the *favela* and during outings into the prejudiced world outside the *favela* (for example, going to the beach or other public spaces elsewhere in the city). Others appreciated having the same group of friends from childhood through adolescence. Overall, this group of young men was an anti-gang gang. They used the language of more violent *bondes* but in fact sought to protect themselves by posturing like a gang to stay out of gang-related and *comando*-related violence.

In all four settings, youth programmes and schools sometimes seek to create or stimulate the formation of alternative, pro-social peer groups – peer groups that do not encourage violence. Religious groups offer this space for some young men, as do sports groups. While male peer groups are often demonized, and often seen as a threat, for many young men they are a tremendous source of support and companionship in the face of material poverty and social exclusion.

The trouble with young men

In examining the multiple ways that structural violence or social exclusion leaves its marks, we see how young men often show anger and mistrust of the middle class; they often internalize some of the negative stereotypes others hold of them. The subtext, the internal dialogue, that many young men in these settings have is: *If you call me nigger, I'll become a nigger – bigger and badder than you imagined. If you think I am a troublemaker or hooligan, wait and see what I can do the next time the riots start. If you think I am a* favelado, *you'll get your due.*[2] Others become unsure of themselves and reluctant to leave the isolated worlds of their low-income neighbourhoods.

The social exclusion described in this chapter must be called violence. It psychologically wounds, materially kills, compromises health and brings truncated life options for children, youth and adults. Chapter 5 will look at how it turns to interpersonal violence for some young men, particularly those who seek out gangs as a way to mitigate a sense of powerlessness and to be part of consumer society. It would be simplistic to say that social exclusion causes such violence. The majority of young people – male and female – in these circumstances do not become involved in gangs or other antisocial activities.

Young women, girls and adult women of course experience tremendous challenges, racism and unequal opportunities in these settings. They endure physical violence from partners and face long hours and low pay, usually working in domestic work or something similar. They face gender-specific challenges that are not highlighted here, but are insidious and life-destroying in their own gendered ways.

As we have seen here, social exclusion psychologically wounds young men in gender-specific ways. The chief mandate of manhood is to earn income, to work, to become financially dependent and to support others, if possible. This income is a prerequisite for attracting young women and being able to form a stable relationship or start a family. To be an out-of-work young man is *not* to be a man, it is to be a boy, to lack status. Indeed, the term 'boy' has historically been hurled as an insult to African male slaves and their male descendants. It is a term that in effect strips them of their manhood, and reminds them of their lack of power in the system. For many young men, to be socially excluded *and* to be denied the title of manhood is injustice squared.

Chapter 5

In the headlines

Interpersonal violence and gang involvement

In Paulo Lin's 1997 book *Cidade de Deus* (City of God), on which the 2002 film of the same name is based, a young man is urged by his male peers to kill a wounded rival gang member. His friends tease him for the fact that he has never killed anyone. Thinking to himself that he wants their respect and consideration, he fires six shots into the wounded rival gang member. The book and film represent a dramitised account of youth and drug trafficking based on actual events in one of Rio de Janeiro's *favelas*. The scene hints at the connection between how manhood is defined and the violence that has come to characterize Rio de Janerio and other parts of the world. Entire books and thousands of articles have been written about factors associated with young men's violence and gang involvement. Here, the focus will be on two issues. The first is: how can non-violence or resistance strategies to violent versions of manhood be promoted in these settings? The second is, what is specifically *male* about this violence?

Giving so much attention to violence may give the impression that all or most low-income, urban-based young men *are* violent, have the potential to be violent or are gang-involved. In fact, it is important that this chapter begins with the following affirmation: in the low-income, urban settings discussed in this book, the vast majority of young men are *not* involved in gangs and do not use serious interpersonal violence against other young men, nor physical violence against their girlfriends and other partners.

That said, violent young men get much more air time and pages devoted to them than their non-violent counterparts. In the United States and in Brazil, books and movies about gang-related violence have captured the public imagination. In 2002–03 in Brazil, the movie *City of God* filled theatres with mostly middle-class audiences. Many residents and community members of the actual neighbourhood (Cidade de Deus) complained about the film. They did not, for the most part, question its historical accuracy. The film portrayed events that happened in the 1980s when many of the contemporary gangs in Rio's *favelas* were forming. What community leaders questioned was the one-sided portrayal of the neighbourhood they call home. Where were the voices for non-violence? Where were the non-violent young men?

One of the bestselling books in Brazil in 2003 was *Abusado* (which might translate as 'the brat'), the story of one of the most flamboyant gang leaders in Rio de Janeiro (Barcellos 2003). Like *City of God*, it was hailed as highly accurate but again, community leaders criticized it for telling only one part of the story. Where are the books and movies about the woman who has cared for several generations of children in her home, or the community leader who negotiates with the city government to bring services to the community? What of the non-violent young men in these settings? Unless they become football stars or musicians, or artists or politicians, they do not make the headlines and their lives do not seem worthy of books and movies.

At times interest and focus on male violence seems to be a form of social pornography – to titillate our fears and give us an adrenaline rush. Just as sexual pornography frequently affirms gender stereotypes, too often, journalistic and film versions of urban violence confirm middle-class stereotypes that young men in low-income communities are violent, and that the best the middle class can do is build more prisons and higher and stronger walls around their homes. An article in one of Brazil's major newspapers reported that a growing number of upper- and middle-income families are constructing fortified 'bunkers' or safe rooms in their apartments and houses, in case of robbery or attack; one company said they had installed 320 such bunkers in homes in São Paulo in the previous three years (O Globo 2004a). This is only one example of the growing, multimillion-dollar private security industry in Brazil and elsewhere in Latin America and the Caribbean.

This is not to deny the existence of the violence that drives middle class fears. As previously discussed, young men are most frequently its victims, but the middle class is also affected. However, in the case of gang-related violence and violence in low-income, urban settings, the stories told are too often one-sided and policies and social practices frequently treat all low-income young men as actual or potential criminals.

Young men and violence

Worldwide, data on violence suggest that young men in the Americas and in some specific countries in sub-Saharan Africa are more likely to kill other young men, and to be killed, than in the rest of the world. The homicide rate in Latin America and the Caribbean is about 20 per 10,000 per year, the highest of any region in the world. The highest rate in the region (and the world) is in fact to be found in Colombia, where between 1991 and 1995, there were 112,000 homicides, of which 41,000 were young people, the vast majority male (Ayres 1998).

The World Health Organization has estimated that in 2000 there were 155,000 deaths worldwide to young men ages 15–29 by homicide, of which close to half, or 72,000, were in the Americas.[1] This means that the risk of dying from homicide for a young man aged 15–29 in the Americas is nearly 28 times higher than the average worldwide risk. Furthermore, the rate of male youth homicide is higher than that of young women everywhere in the world, and the ratio of male–female homicide rates tends to be higher in those countries with higher rates of male homicide (WHO 2002).

In the Caribbean, 80 per cent of violent crimes are carried out by men, usually younger men. Similarly, in the rest of the world, some 90 per cent of lethal violence is committed by men, usually younger men, and nearly two-thirds of this violence is committed against other young men (Archer 1994). Homicide is the third leading cause of death in men aged 10–19 in the United States and accounted for 42 per cent of deaths among young black males from 1980 to 1990 (US Department of Health and Human Services 1991). Data from Rio de Janeiro in 1995 confirmed that 91 per cent of the city's homicide victims were male, and 57 per cent were between the ages of 15 and 29 (Moser and van Bronkhorst 1999).

Clearly, homicide is not the only form of young men's violence, although it is the form most often counted consistently across countries. Other forms of violence – fighting, vandalism, assaults, gender-based or dating violence – are more common and affect many more young people than do homicide. Studies of non-fatal violence suggest that for every homicide, there are between 20 and 40 victims of other forms of violence who seek hospital treatment (WHO 2002). The majority of the victims are male, except when it comes to domestic violence.

In various studies around the world, about one-third of young people say they have been involved in fighting, with boys two to three times as likely to report being involved in fights when compared to girls (WHO 2002). The personal story I related of having got involved in a fight with another boy over a girl when I was 10 plays outside-out in similar ways but often with more serious consequences in thousands of schoolyards and neighbourhoods everyday around the world. In a study of youth in the Western Cape Region of South Africa, for example, 9.8 per cent of boys and 1.3 per cent of girls interviewed in secondary schools reported having carried knives to school in the previous month (WHO 2002).

Violence and its public costs consume up to 15 per cent of the gross national products of some countries. One study suggests that Colombia's per capita income might be one-third higher now if not for the high rates of violence and crime since the late 1980s (Ayres 1998). In Rio de Janeiro, the total economic cost in 1993 from violence was estimated at US$1 billion.

Interpersonal violence manifests itself in other ways as well. As of 2002, 20 of 53 countries in the African continent had some ongoing armed conflict. Many if not most of the estimated 300,000 child soldiers (under age 18) worldwide are found in the region (Verhey 2001). There is relatively little discussion of gender in studies on child soldiers, and when there is it focuses on girls. In conflict settings such as these, girls are more likely to serve supporting roles, and are too often victims of sexual violence carried out by these armed men and boys. Boys, who represent the vast majority of child soldiers, are often trained in killing and sexually abusing, forced to kill and face other traumatic experiences in witnessing or being victimized in conflict settings.

To these examples, one could add armed vigilante groups in parts of Nigeria, or gangs in urban areas in South Africa. Nonetheless, there has been little discussion of how boys are raised in these settings, and in reports about this violence, or what is gender-specific about this violence. The availability of thousands of young men with limited or no access to mean-ingful employment, few other sources of identity and socialized into rigid views and violent versions of manhood has played directly into the hands of local and national warlords and vigilante groups. It is convenient, for example, that Charles Taylor in Liberia and rebel leaders in Sierra Leone had at their disposal thousands of young men (many of whom had wit-nessed other young men kill their own family members, others who were coerced into combatant roles). These are boys and young men who are socialized into gender-ordered pathways that include the use of violence and cruelty against other men, and sexual violence against girls and women. The different armed groups in Liberia and Sierra Leone had specific ways of brutalizing young men into becoming killers, but this particular form of socialization happened in settings that already supported male violence generally.

In Nigeria, young men, usually low-income young men, are those most likely to be on the front line of violence between Christian and Muslim groups – violence that has resulted in thousands of deaths and continues to be a source of concern in the country. The violence against international oil companies in the Delta region of Nigeria has also been mostly perpetrated by young men. As happens in many parts of the world, once groups of young men are armed and encouraged to use these weapons, what starts as politically focused violence can turn into general hooliganism and harassment.

Gangs that once mostly or only attacked oil company staff and their installations now create havoc in some major cities in the region. Vigilante groups, one of the most famous being the Bakassi Boys, were initially started as self-defence groups set up to protect market sellers from robbery; they are now subsidized by the government as an explicit public security project. The Bakassi Boys currently wield tremendous extrajudicial power in parts of Nigeria and carry out summary executions at the whim of local politicians. They have probably reduced crime in some cities (if we do not count their own vigilante activity as a crime). But they also kill human rights activists or whoever dares to speak out against them (Human Rights Watch/Centre for Law Enforcement 2002).

Much of the homicide among young men is related to gang activity; indeed most male antisocial behaviour and interpersonal violence (outside the home) takes place in a group setting, much of that as part of organized gangs. In Nicaragua, for example, almost half of all crime and delinquency is said to be related to gangs (Rodgers 1999). In the Western Cape Region of South Africa, 90,000 young people are reported to be members of gangs. In El Salvador, some 30,000–35,000 young people are said to participate in gangs. In the United States, researchers estimate that there are 31,000 gangs in 4800 cities across the country. A WHO (2002) study found that among 1,000 young people interviewed in a low-income urban area, 30 per cent were involved in gangs, and those who were involved in gangs accounted for 70 per cent of self-reported violent crimes in the sample (WHO 2002).

To be sure, there are tremendous differences in the nature of gang activity in the regions discussed here, but there are also commonalities. Gang members are overwhelmingly low-income young men who project specific versions of manhood associated with violence, attracting women and acquiring consumer goods and status through the use of violence.

Theories on violence

But what causes interpersonal violence? And why do some young men use violence and get involved in gangs and others do not? Much of the research on violence and delinquency in the United States and Western Europe has sought to identify early childhood predictors of violent behaviour (including biologically based tendencies, such as temperament, aggressiveness and hyperactivity). Overall, these biological or temperamental based predictors of later violent behaviour for young men are relatively weak in their explanatory power. Many authors have concluded that while there may be some evidence for the early propensity of aggression in boys, the majority of violent behaviour is explained by social factors during adolescence and childhood. In other words, boys are not born violent – they learn to be violent. And they mainly learn to be violent by seeing other boys and men use violence, by witnessing violence, by themselves being victims of violence in the home, at school and in their neighbourhoods and by seeing violence as an effective means to acquire income, power and respect and attract women.[2]

Violence is not caused by poverty; the violence I witnessed in my middle-class high school was not in a context of poverty, nor were the infamous school shootings in Columbine, Colorado in 1999. But interpersonal violence does flourish in conditions of poverty and social exclusion. More important than poverty, though, is the issue of income inequality. Violence seems to be the highest in those settings where too few wealthy individuals control the lion's share of goods and resources and the poor majority have access to less than their share. It is no statistical accident that the United States and the United Kingdom have among the highest rates of violence among industrialized countries; they also have among the worst income distribution among higher-income countries. Similarly, the countries with the highest rates of violence in Latin America and the Caribbean also have some of the worst income distribution patterns in the world, as does South Africa. In short, frustration and anger over an unequal distribution of opportunities are the breeding grounds for violence, rather than abject poverty per se.

Various studies confirm that violence and gang involvement are highest in countries and cities where community cohesion has broken down, or social institutions (the family, religious groups, schools, the workplace) have become stressed (Rodgers 1999). Indeed, gangs and other forms of organized violence become attractive in such settings, precisely when families and other social institutions have little relevance to young men's lives or are not able to help them fulfil what they perceive are the mandates of manhood – namely to acquire income, status and attract women. A WHO review of violence data worldwide concludes that violence is higher in countries undergoing rapid change (WHO 2002). Where the rule of law does not exist or is fragile, where opportunities for employment are blocked and when individuals experience frustration on a large scale, interpersonal violence – mostly carried out by young men – increases. But, as mentioned in Chapter 1, it still generally involves only a minority of young men.

At the level of the family, in situations of social exclusion and stress, low-income families often have a reduced ability to effectively monitor the behaviour and whereabouts of their sons (and daughters) in appropriate ways. Stressed parents in low-income settings often use coercive, physical discipline against children, and more often with boys than with girls. They generally have good intentions, and may be trying as best they understand to keep their sons (and daughters) safe and out of gangs or away from gang-related violence. In low-income communities around the world, mothers can be seen aggressively treating young children who have wandered outside the house. In one incident witnessed in one such setting, a mother who hit her wayward child explained that she had to 'teach him to stay inside, or he'll get hurt. The bullets can start flying anytime.' Stressed parents in such settings often face challenges in keeping their children, but particularly their sons, safe from the violence around them. Others lack the energy and time to engage their sons in meaningful discussions about their expectations of them and their concerns for their safety. The father of one young man interviewed said he would venture out into the community at two or three o'clock in the morning to find his son, but few parents in such stressed situations have this energy.

Some researchers suggest that boys living in violent neighbourhoods and households learn that violence is a way to resolve conflicts, are often not exposed to other ways of resolving conflicts and, in turn, use the violence they learned in their homes to resolve conflicts outside their homes. Some work in the United States suggests that violent and delinquent boys, when compared to less-violent and non-delinquent control groups, are more likely to perceive or attribute hostile intent in the actions of others (McAlister 1998). Boys who use violence have learned that individuals in their immediate environment often have hostile intentions toward them – including members of their own family – and thus these young men may inappropriately attribute hostile intent in others even when none may exist. In other words, boys who use violence may have shorter fuses and see the world as a mostly hostile place.

The male peer group is also a factor in violent and delinquent behaviour. Studies of delinquency in Western Europe and the United States suggest a pattern in which a relatively small number of males (generally in low-income urban settings) commit a few delinquent acts, are subsequently labelled and eventually accept and internalize the label and identity of delinquent. Such behaviours start early in childhood and are strongly related to the peer group, that is associating with a peer group that encouraged violence (Elliott 1994). We should be careful, however, not to demonize male peer groups. Some encourage fighting, sexual conquests and violent versions of manhood, but others encourage the opposite. For some young men, as previously discussed, the male peer group can be a place to reinforce a non-violent identity and to cope with the violence around them.

Labelling young men as violent is also a major contributor to violence. Earlier in this chapter, I criticized the one-sided images of young men from *favelas* in recent books and films. This criticism is not gratuitous; it is grounded in the fact that these labels and stereotypes affect the lives of individuals in direct and real ways. Low-income young men who have heard from teachers, parents, the media and the world around them that they are violent are more likely to become violent. Young men who have been frequently and falsely accused of violence, like the examples seen of police accusations and harassment, may be more likely to use violence.

To offer one example, during one visit to a public school in Rio de Janeiro, a teacher pointed out one young man and said: 'His brother is in the *comando*. I have my eye on him. He may go the same way.' The young man in question squirmed in his seat and spoke with others while the teacher was talking, but then so were half of the children in the classroom. These labels often become self-fulfilling prophecies, creating anger and resentment on the part of young men – anger that may turn into violence. One young man in Jamaica said this, with clear anger in his voice:

> You get labelled 'inner city' . . . 'ghetto'. A 'ghetto' – nobody even knows what that means! Bob Marley and a lot of intelligent guys come from places that

they [the middle class] call ghettos. There are lawyers and doctors who live
in ghettos. A lot of people think that the ghetto is only crime and violence
and drugs. Yes, you have that . . . you have people killing to survive. Some
youth get involved in posses [youth gangs] and drug dealing just to have
somebody to talk to.

(Out-of-school youth, 22, Kingston, Jamaica)

For many low-income young men, labelling and stereotypes reduce the mar-
gin they have to make mistakes, particularly in an era where 'zero tolerance'
has become an international tendency. For many low-income young men,
this means that any involvement in fights or disruptive behaviour can begin
a cycle of exclusion, expulsion and punishment. Studies confirm that boys
who have attention deficit problems or other school behaviour problems
are more likely to later use violent behaviour. However, attention deficit
problems do not cause violent behaviour. Instead, parents and teachers
often label these behaviours as troublesome and react in authoritarian or
controlling ways (Sampson and Laub 1993). The cycle often goes like this:
a boy acts out in a minor way, but is punished disproportionately for his
actions. Chafing at this discipline, he acts out even more, and the punishment the next time around is even more severe, causing him to act out again
– in even more dangerous ways.

Violence can also be a form of self-protection, both physical protection –
protecting one's own body – as well as psychological protection. Research
has found a survival and instrumental function of violence for young men
in low-income communities. For many low-income males, many of whom
have little else which gives them meaning and clear roles in society, violence
can also be a way of maintaining status in the male peer group and of
preventing violence against oneself (Schwartz 1987; Anderson 1990;
Majors and Billson 1993; Archer 1994).

A 'bad boy' instils fear and wields power. He steps out from his
anonymity and gets attention; even if that attention is negative, he is seen.
During one group discussion in Rio de Janeiro, a gang-involved young man
came into the session and asked what was going on. He had a pistol at his
waist and was pleased with the fact that he could disrupt the session and
scare everyone present. He helped himself to the restroom in the meeting
facility, and while there, the group activity stopped. No one said a word.
Then he left with a sneer, apparently pleased with the power he could wield
over 25 other young men. Compare this display of bravado with the
previous example described of powerlessness that João faced when he
confronted police repression or callous middle-class customers.

Nicholas Emler and Stephen Reicher (1995) have suggested that violence
and antisocial behaviour for many adolescent males is a deliberate 'reputa-
tional project', an effort to affirm an identity to others as delinquent or violent in order to fit in the antisocial peer group – particularly for those young

men who see mainstream goals and identities as beyond their reach (or who feel they have been rejected by mainstream social institutions). Given that most delinquent behaviour happens in groups and that most delinquent acts are committed by a relatively small number of young men, it seems reasonable to conclude that violent and antisocial behaviour is frequently an expression of a certain form of identity. Young men who cannot get attention for other qualities or achieve identity through other means may find that being a 'tough guy' is better than going unnoticed. Acts that are labelled by teachers and parents as a risky or antisocial behaviour may be ways for the individual to prove himself or become part of a group, or simply to be recognized for something.

The case of Murilo

A young man named Murilo, who was interviewed in Rio de Janeiro, offers a useful case study for how these issues interact. Murilo was 17 when the interviews began. He is African Brazilian, large in stature, clowns and jokes frequently, and can also be moody or impulsive, closing off to himself, or walking away from a group activity in anger. He has occasional outbursts when he may yell at a peer, or at a coordinator of the group about something he does not agree with. He is also thoughtful, reflective and able to engage in conversations with adults with ease, including international visitors and representatives of the government agency that funded some of our work.

Murilo came from a family of mother, father and a younger brother. This was a somewhat unusual arrangement in Maré, considering the large number of mother-only households and the number of households involving a second marriage or union and children from previous unions. Both of Murilo's parents work in low-level administrative positions in government agencies.

Murilo reported having an extremely tense relationship with his parents, particularly with his mother. On occasional visits to his house, his mother was observed being verbally aggressive with him, and he was sometimes verbally aggressive back to her. Both in Murilo's presence and when he was not around, his parents said that he was a difficult child; I heard few positive words spoken directly to him by his parents. His mother showed considerable negative affect toward him:

> he was a boy who was always so calm – huh! – that at the age of 1 day old he already rolled around in bed. At 3 months he already a tooth, and he walked at 9 months. He started off running from the beginning. He always had too much energy for my liking . . . He has always been very, very, very tiring.
>
> (Murilo's mother)

Although Murilo was clearly intelligent, he had had frequent problems at school and had been expelled from three different schools. During one of those expulsions, his parents said they thought that he was 'crazy' and sent him to see a psychologist. His father said this of him:

> I don't trust Murilo. If I could trust Murilo, I could live with all the rest . . . If Murilo told me where he really was going to be . . . but Murilo tells you he will be someplace and he's not there. I'm tired of him. I've been battling this since he was 6 years old. . . When he was little, he humiliated the janitor at his school. [Murilo was involved in a prank with a younger boy] and when the janitor took him to the principal's office, Murilo told him [the janitor] that he was a [bumpkin], who didn't have an education, who was starving and poor, and said 'my father pays your salary, remember that' . . . Can you imagine that? . . . He was 9 or 10 when that happened.
>
> (Murilo's father)

Pranks, fights, disruptive behaviour and challenging authority figures are fairly routine for many adolescents and children. Learning limits, for many children, requires testing these limits. If a middle-class young person spoke rudely to school staff, it would likely result in a reprimand, not expulsion.

In many ways, acting out and being troublesome seems to have become Murilo's identity; others see him that way, so he goes with it. He said that in his last school, he was not getting in as much trouble because he did not have an 'audience' that expected him to act out: 'Going to a school where you don't know anyone is better. I get in more trouble when I know everyone.' Perhaps he 'gets in trouble' because his close friends and peers expect him to act out, and he feels he has to play the role for which he has become known.

Teachers, adults who worked with him and his own parents saw Murilo as out-of-control and aggressive. To me, however, Murilo seemed bored most of the time. I had the chance to interact with him in out-of-school time, away from his parents, in activities that he enjoyed and helped construct. He was a singer, dancer and songwriter (he wrote rap songs, including some about non-violence). He was full of ideas and questions about the world. He was offended and angered by injustice and immediately spoke back when he felt an injustice had been committed. Some psychologists and his parents might want to give him the label of 'troublesome', or dress up this label by calling him hyperactive. I thought that Murilo needed more stimulation and challenges – including a classroom setting that could make learning come to life rather than focusing on making him sit still. For a time, he was a dancer in an African Brazilian dance troupe. He performed as one of the lead dancers in several dozen performances. During that time, he seemed the calmest and most focused I had seen him.

Almost two years after I first met Murilo, he was arrested. He had friends in the *comando*, and a family friend who was part of it. He sometimes bragged of hanging out with gang members. However, he did not seem to have the disposition to participate in selling drugs or carrying weapons. It seemed that he just hung out with them, telling his non-gang peers about it, perhaps as a way to maintain his 'bad guy' reputation. Perhaps it was part youthful invincibility that he thought he could hang out with gang members but stay out of trouble. His parents hired a lawyer to defend him, and we wrote letters for him, testifying that this was his first offence and that he was part of a community programme. As a result, he got off with a short probation.

A short time later, his parents helped him find a job as a janitor at one of Rio's public universities. After having seen Murilo perform before an audience, it seemed out of place to see him hauling a broom and dressed in the uniform of a janitorial staff. He seemed bored, although he apparently wanted us to think that all was okay.

To be a black man carrying a broom at a large public university in Brazil, where the vast majority of students are white and middle class, is to be invisible. It was no surprise when a few months later he was arrested again in similar circumstances – hanging out with known drug dealers in a stolen car with guns. This time, now an adult, he received a five-year prison sentence.

While presented in brief here, Murilo's story highlights the complex interactions that can lead to antisocial behaviour and gang involvement. It illustrates a cycle of negative affect from parents, combined with labelling on the part of teachers and parents, and the lack of sustained activities and options to engage energetic and ambitious young men like Murilo. His parents could not discipline nor set limits for Murilo without being aggressive, which in turn pushed Murilo to respond aggressively. Clearly, his parents meant well for him. They themselves had struggled financially and wanted him to have even more opportunities – to be better off than they were.

Murilo may have had some emotional and learning problems. He may have had difficulties sitting still, but he was clearly able to concentrate – when there was something that grabbed his attention. There are also peer group issues involved. While Murilo had mostly non-gang peers, the fact that he interacted with friends who were part of the *comando* increased the chance that he would get involved in some way or that he would be in the wrong place when violence broke out.

We also see in Murilo's case and others, that violence is often a part of male identity. For young men living in a setting like a *favela* in Rio de Janeiro, violence can also serve an instrumental, survival function. Indeed, the Brazilian anthropologist Alba Zaluar (1994) suggests that young men who participate in *comandos* in *favelas* buy into or are socialized into a 'warrior ethos', an identity and set of codes which involves, among other things, a willingness to use violence to achieve one's goals, including having access to consumer goods. Projecting the *bandido* identity – even if only occasionally – was a source of status for Murilo.

All this suggests that solutions to violence and violence prevention with young men will have to be multifaceted. No single programme or policy – gun control or midnight sports activities – will by themselves resolve the problem. If individual, community, peer group, family and structural issues are involved in the problem, they must also be invoked for the solution.

Why young men join gangs

Although their activities and rituals may differ widely, gangs are prevalent in various parts of the world, in addition to settings like Murilo's neighbourhood in Brazil. There are reports of gangs in Central America, Mexico, Colombia, the Caribbean, parts of Africa, India and parts of Europe. Armed groups of young men, as previously mentioned, are terrorizing parts of the Delta region in Nigeria. In South Africa, groups of young men – some of whom were once militants in the ANC – have formed armed gangs that rob and kidnap. Gang behaviour has been widely studied in the United States as well. In the case of Chicago, where I spoke with both gang-involved and non-gang-involved young men, there were an estimated 40 major street gangs active, each responsible for at least 1000 police-recorded criminal incidents between 1987 and 1990; in 1990 Chicago police estimated that 40,000 youth were involved in gangs (Block and Block 1995).

In most settings, gang-involved youth are a minority of young people, although a small minority can wreck havoc on communities. For example, a study on drug-trafficking gangs in Rio de Janeiro asserted that 12,527 children aged 8–18 in the city participate in drug-trafficking activities – 5773 of those between the ages of 15 and 17. In the same age range, only 3200 youth aged 15–17 are employed in other professions. If these data are correct, drug trafficking employs more young men aged 15–17 in low-income areas in Rio de Janeiro than do conventional forms of employment (O Globo 2002b). This same study concluded that 1.03 per cent of youth from *favelas* work in drug trafficking. Similarly, in a study sponsored by the International Labour Office (ILO), 5000 to 6000 youth in Rio de Janeiro were estimated to be participating in drug-trafficking gangs, representing only about 0.3 per cent of the total youth (15–24) population in the city, and 1.5 per cent of the total youth population living in low-income areas in the city (Souza and Urani 2002). In either case, the actual number of young men who participate in gang-related activity is relatively small, but the gang-associated version of manhood has implications beyond this membership.

Why do young men join gangs? Previous chapters have already included some examples and insights on this, but it is useful to offer more detail. We see in the discourses and life stories of young men in these settings that, faced with a shortage of stable and viable employment, gang involvement, particularly when it involves drug trafficking, has become a vocational alternative for some young men, who often face family and social pressure to drop out of school at early ages to work.

Participating in gangs is a mostly male phenomenon that generally implies projecting or adhering to a specific version of masculinity characterized by:

- the use of armed violence to achieve one's goals, and a willingness to kill if necessary
- callous attitudes toward women, including violence against women
- an exaggerated sense of male honour and a propensity to use violence in minor altercations and insults.

Of course, other young men not participating in gangs in various parts of the world may similarly adhere to some or all of these values. Indeed, some authors suggest that this version of masculinity reinforced by gangs represents an extreme or exaggerated version of a prevailing or hegemonic masculinity found in low-income settings in Brazil (Zaluar 1994). In the case of Rio de Janeiro, to be a *bandido* – a member of the *comandos* – is to be in many ways a standard-bearer of the most visible and fear-inspiring version of what it means to be a man. Active *comando* members are generally always men, and usually young men.[3]

An ILO study in Brazil confirmed that being in a *comando* provides status and access to consumer goods for those young men involved. Based on interviews with young men involved, the authors conclude that

> outlaw activities are a concrete life and survival alternative, regardless of the risk entailed. . . In this context, submission becomes even more humiliating. Children and young adults seek autonomy, adrenaline, independence and power, which are essentially expressed by their image and perceived by their peers.
>
> (Souza and Urani 2002: 14)

In summary, young men interviewed for the ILO study justified their participation in the *comandos* for three main reasons: money, women and respect.

It seems reasonable to assert that the vast majority of (heterosexual) young men in low-income settings around the world want money, women and respect. As we saw earlier, these are the main mandates of heterosexual versions of manhood. What sets the young men in gangs and *comandos* apart is the means they are willing to use (or have at hand) to acquire these things. In their quest for money, women and respect, gang-involved young men display extreme or exaggerated versions of traditional masculinity.

How young men in gangs and *comandos* treat their female partners is illustrative of this point. The ILO study in Brazil reported that 22.5 per cent of young men interviewed who were involved in the *comandos* were married or in a stable union. This is higher than rates of marriage for young men in the same age range, suggesting that the income from drug trafficking allows young men to have access to female partners and form families earlier than their non-gang-involved peers. As João said: 'A hard worker can go months without a girlfriend, but a *bandido* [member of the drug-trafficking *comando*] always has two or three women.' Being a *bandido* means having several female partners and being able to demand absolute loyalty from them. A young woman connected to a *comando* member, even after she has broken off from him, cannot be seen with another man in the community. And if she were to sexually betray him while he was imprisoned, she would likely be killed.

Similar attitudes can be seen in the discourses of young men in the Caribbean and the United States. One gang-involved young man in Chicago showed a callous attitude toward girls and hinted at the transactional nature of male–female relationships in the context of gang involvement:

> Girls! They're like, they sit in front of your face and get one of those sad looks and then they say 'there ain't nothin' to do, let's go out.' I went out with this girl a couple of days ago [to 'go out' implied a date and having sex] and she wanted to go out again [right after that]. And she told me she wanted these new shoes and I told her that I ain't got enough money for that. That would be like my whole paycheck right there . . . from the money I get [from his work with a gang]. They just want you to spend all your money . . . [Just because I am in a gang] they think I'm a money man.
>
> (Davin, 15, African American, Chicago)

What about the importance of income derived from drug trafficking? In 2002, young people involved with the *comandos* in Rio de Janeiro said they earned between R$240 and R$320 (between US$87 and US$116) a month as informants up to R$1200 (about US$430) for 'sales managers' (O Globo 2002b). Compare this to the fact that household monthly per capita earnings at the same time were R$134 (about US$48) in low income neighbourhoods compared to city average of about R$700 (about US$250) (Souza and Urani 2002).

However, possibly even more important than income is status. As seen in Chapters 1 and 2, the chief mandate of manhood in most of the world is to acquire work and income. And, if male identity is defined by work, having stable employment (legal or illegal) that offers respect *and* income is central to achieving status. Murilo described the situation thus:

GB: What does it mean [for a man] to work?
MURILO: You have to work. Because you want to have your [own] things and at least when you're 20 or 25, you want your things organized . . . together [have a family and support yourself]. And if you don't work, you're gonna have to rob to make a living. You're not going to be [as

a man], walking around with nothing to do or wear. I prefer to work [than to steal].

Not to have work and the income and status associated, as these young men suggest, is to be a 'nobody', to lack status before one's family, potential and actual female partners, one's peers and society in general. Beyond income, being in gangs can bring respect on other fronts. For young men who have few other sources of being socially recognized, being tough or an 'outlaw' may be all there is. Other young men may join gangs for protection or for a sense of belonging. When asked why young men join gangs, one young man in Chicago said:

> For protection. They [those who get involved in gangs] are scared. Like [somebody] may approach them and they don't got nobody on their side to help them with the gangs. Some just do gangs because they feel lost, like if something happened to someone in their family they just don't know how to handle it.
>
> (Johnny, 18, African American, Chicago)

Family stress is also a factor involved in gang involvement. Several of the young men in the Caribbean, Brazil and the United States who had participated in gangs showed family-related difficulties. One young man, as previously mentioned, said he was the only living male in his family. Other young men reported family violence – particularly violence by a stepfather or father against a mother – or a substance use problem in the family. Young men in Rio de Janeiro who became involved in gangs reported having spent time working and/or living on the streets. This experience, particularly of having to sell on the streets, was seen as degrading. Selling candy on the streets or on a bus, or selling water at intersections, for example, were seen as desperation, not as jobs that provided a solid sense of identity and respect. In this context, invitations from gang-involved friends or colleagues became attractive. For some young men, gang involvement was the only stable employment they had ever had:

GB: You said you were 10 years old when you left school and went to work on the street?

GINALDO: We were hard up . . . that's why I stopped going to school [and went to work on the street]. I need to get some money to buy anything I could for our house. My father abandoned us. I was hungry . . . we went to bed hungry, woke up hungry. So I went to the street to get for money . . . to shine shoes . . .

GB: And how did you get involved in the *comandos*?

GINALDO: It [the invitation to join] was from a guy who worked in drug sales . . . he asked me if I wanted to manage the sales and I said yes, and so I managed it . . . I said, shit, I'm going to work. I got myself a job!

It is striking that the excitement in his voice suggests the same kind of pride or satisfaction when a young man acquires his first job in conventional employment.

Why most young men stay out of gangs

It is important not to overstate the power of gangs. Clearly for some young men, gangs are a powerful pull to achieve a visible, male identity, find a sense of belonging, attract women and acquire income. But the majority of young men find ways to stay out of gangs – even those who are brothers, friends or classmates of gang members. Many of the young men interviewed in Chicago and Rio de Janeiro said that gangs had never approached them. Some said they believed the gangs left them alone because they kept to themselves, or in some way made it known that they were not interested and were not appropriate gang material – they did not have the 'disposition'.

In the case of Chicago, while some young men told of having been pressured or invited to be in gangs, or having been in gangs, others found it fairly easy to stay out of gangs. For some young men, this meant projecting an identity of being a good student, being seen as too shy or weak, having strong religious affiliations, or having a strong or outgoing personality that enabled them to be friends with gang members (and receive the protection from being associated with gang members) without having to be a fully fledged member of the gang. However, even for those young men who did not feel direct pressure from gangs and who did not accept this gang-related version of manhood, gangs nonetheless are a powerful source of norms and identity that nearly all the young men had to contend with, even if only to reject.

For some young men, gang-related violence seemed absurd, even silly. Some young men told of being approached by friends in gangs, but felt confident in turning them away. One young man in Chicago, named Anthony, was part of a special leadership programme at his school and quite articulate. He considered himself, and others saw him, as an informal counsellor; he was frequently sought out for advice and for some students, was seen as a useful intermediary to talk to teachers. Anthony played US football and had shoulders and a physique that gangs wanted on their side, and which could be seen as threatening to some adults. He described himself as a Christian and as actively religious. To diffuse the fact that some adults felt threatened by his muscular build (and simply for being a young African American man), he had a cross with the word 'Jesus' written above it tattooed on one of his triceps. Even on cold winter days in Chicago, Anthony frequently had his shirt sleeves rolled up so the tattoo could be seen. When I asked Anthony about gangs he replied as follows:

GB: Have gangs approached you?

ANTHONY: Oh, all the time. You know they . . . say things like 'Tone, why don't you come home?' [meaning become part of the gang in the building where you live] and I respond to them in a sarcastic way but I mean it, like 'I'm already home' . . . but I strongly . . . believe that I know that I will never be part of such organization [a gang] even though I live around them . . . I mean I get along real well with them. There's no problem at all . . .

GB: And so when you joke with them and say 'You're the one who needs to come home' do they back off?

ANTHONY: Yes, I mean they immediately [back off], it's like I got the picture, I understand, they leave it alone.

For many young men, family ties were reported to be the reason they stayed out of gangs. Those who got involved with gangs in Chicago and Rio de Janeiro were described by some non-gang-involved young men as 'having nothing to lose' by joining. On the other hand, those who stayed out of gangs showed concern over how a parent or family member would react if they became involved in a gang. One young man from Chicago said:

LIONEL: I not like a gangbanger because of the way my mother raised me. I am scared, you know. It's like it's different things you don't do, especially when you know somebody loves [you] and you don't have to do those things and you don't have to turn to the streets. I have a strong family.

GB: When you say you're scared, scared of what?

LIONEL: My mother getting on me. And in one more year I will be 18 and I know for sure that my Mom will put me out [of the house] if I screw up. My Mom is not that type of person that would want a lot of pressure on her. Because bills are enough for her. It certain things that you wouldn't do to my mother and certain things my mother wouldn't let you do to her.

Lionel also showed another quality that enabled many young men to stay out of gangs – having some other identity or ability. In his case, he was a disk jockey (DJ), and apparently good at it:

GB: How did you react to gangs in your neighbourhood?

LIONEL: By me getting into music and by me being the person able to stand up for myself, that gave me a good reputation . . . just being the person

I am. People go crazy over a DJ. They like to know someone . . . you know, like a celebrity.

Another factor in staying out of gangs, or getting out for those involved, was fear of death or injury. Many young men are openly scared of gang-related violence, as will be seen later. In most settings, being a man generally means not being afraid, and young men sometimes seemed reluctant to admit their fear; some denied it. But clearly fear is a major motivating factor for staying out of gangs, and for getting out of gangs. Anderson, whose story will be told in more detail later on, had been involved in a gang, but got out when he began to fear for his life:

ANDERSON: I mean I wasn't always outside [the *comandos*] like this. When I dropped out of school, there were some times when I was involved [with the *comando*] and I saw that it wasn't good . . . You go to see a friend, and you see that friend turn against you. You have risks all around you, like them [the *comando*] wanting to get rid of you, or the police. So I thought to myself, am I gonna want this life? Like not being able to sleep a peaceful night? I mean I still have my mother and my grandmother. I don't have my father, but I have my mother, my grandmother, so that's why [I got out] . . .

GB: Tell me more about how you got out of the *comando*.

ANDERSON: . . . everything started to go wrong. The head guy of the *comando* died. And then they tried to kill this young guy who took his place because he was only 17, you know, the others thought they could take over since he was only a kid. And I thought if they try to get rid of him, they're gonna try to get rid of me. So I left and never went back.

Living and coping with interpersonal violence

What is it like to be surrounded by this kind of violence? In the time that I have been working with young men in various low-income communities in Rio de Janeiro, during several moments they have referred to the drug-related violence in their communities as 'this war' or in some way compared the situation to a war.[4] While this comparison may be exaggerated, the ongoing violence that plagues Rio de Janeiro's *favelas* (and comparable communities in places like Kingston, Jamaica, Medellín, Colombia, Chicago, United States, among others) *feels* to many young people (and adults) who live in it, like a war. In all of these settings, as in Rio de Janeiro, it is only a minority of young men who participate in this violence, and are victimized by it, but many young people in these communities have felt or witnessed the violence, as the following narratives illustrate:

> He [the member of the rival *comando*] was chasing after us on a horse . . .
> he was going to kill us . . . There were three of us, my brother and I and
> another guy [who was involved in the *comando*]. He was after my brother
> first, but my brother got away. Then he was after me and I ran to our house
> and hid inside . . . then my brother got there . . . he [the member of the rival
> *comando*] started to beat up my brother . . . beat the shit out of him. The
> next day we found out that the other boy [the brother's friend who was in
> the *comando*] was dead. This guy [from the rival *comando*] killed him.
>
> (Pedro, 17, African Brazilian, Rio de Janeiro)

Another young man who had friends in the *comando* told this story:

> One time . . . some of them [members of the *comando*] slept at my house
> . . . my mother knew them. One of them was like my brother . . . so then one
> day, he and four other friends of his who were in the *comando* slept at our
> house [sleeping at different residences is sometimes utilized as a way to
> avoid police and rival *comandos*] . . . And this day I woke up . . . police
> knocked on the door and I heard them say: 'We have them all, they're here.'
> The guys in our house were armed, right . . . So the police said: 'Open up.'
> And the guys said: 'No, if you come in we'll start shooting' . . . [the police
> caught one of them and] started to beat him and one cop was shooting right
> at him [point blank] . . . this really bad cop . . . Then another police officer
> came and said: 'He's alive. Let's take him to the hospital.' But then this bad
> cop, he said: 'Take him to the hospital? Why? . . . I know this guy . . . 'So then
> they shot at him until he wasn't breathing any more.
>
> (Andre, 16, African Brazilian, Rio de Janeiro)

Similarly, in the United States, studies suggest that while delinquent and
gang-involved males may be a minority, the violence they perpetuate (and
are victims of) has widespread effects and is nearly universally felt. Bell and
Jenkins (1993), in interviews with high school students in south Chicago,
found that more than half had witnessed a beating, more than one-third
had witnessed a robbery, more than half knew someone who had been
robbed, and nearly one-fifth had themselves been victims of robbery. In this
same study, nearly one-fifth said they themselves had pulled a knife, and
nearly 10 per cent said they had stabbed someone.

Young Hispanic boys (ages 11–14) interviewed in Chicago suggested that
violence in the community, and its effects, had reached a certain level of
banality. Two boys in one group had been victims of stabbing and gunshots.
One boy related having been the victim of a gunshot wound three years
before the interview (in a gang-related shooting). He told his story of being
shot in a group setting with a smile and a laugh, almost as if it were a badge
of honour – or perhaps that he had worked hard to hide any fear or trauma
related to it. During some group discussions, both in Chicago and Rio de

Janeiro, when the theme of community violence was introduced, the young men talked over themselves offering incidents they had witnessed or knew of. Several boys seemed to try to tell the goriest story they had ever heard, for example of rival gang members shooting off the testicle of another for revenge. While these perhaps were exaggerations, many of the examples were no doubt true. When asked how this violence made them feel, there was a collective silence in the room until one boy (in a discussion group with Hispanic young men) finally said: 'It [the violence] becomes like a daily thing . . . like once a week you see something or hear something. You're not scared. It's like you just get used to it.'

In such settings, young men feel helpless to protect themselves and their families. They told of getting down on the floor, stepping away from the window, and avoiding places where gang members hang out as among their strategies for physically surviving. But what of the psychological impact? Part of avoiding gangs is also about avoiding eye contact, pretending you do not see, looking down at the ground and keeping quiet. One researcher called the youth who avoided gangs the 'hidden ones' – they tried hard not to be seen, not to call attention to themselves and hoped in the process that gangs, police and other potential threats would leave them alone (Linhales Barker 1995).

All of these survival tactics are psychologically wearing and not very useful for succeeding in other realms, such as the workplace or the school. When you have spent much of your childhood trying *not* to be seen, it is difficult to come into the spotlight and express yourself. Indeed, the cautious, inward-looking and shell-shocked attitudes that many young people in such settings display are not useful for acquiring and taking advantage of opportunities in school, the community and in the workplace.

Ethnicity and violence

Many of the examples included regarding violence up until now have come from Brazil and the United States, with a few from the Caribbean, and have been related to gangs, but violence among young men in some parts of the world plays out across ethnic and religious lines. To offer one example, in Kaduna, in the middle belt region of Nigeria – halfway between the Muslim-majority north and the Christian-majority south – clashes have been frequent between Christian and Muslim young men. Major riots took place in Kaduna in 1987 and again in 1999 around the time that a Miss Universe contest was going to be held in Nigeria. Tensions continue to be high even after the 1999 event, particularly as Muslim leaders have sought to introduce Sharia law in parts of northern Nigeria. Many young men and some staff at youth organizations say they believe that riots of the dimension of the 1999 clashes – that left perhaps as many as 2000 dead – would be unlikely to happen again; however, they said this on the same day that riots took place again, when Christian youths attacked a Mosque and Muslim youths reacted by attacking and damaging some churches.

While the backdrop for ethnic-related violence in Nigeria differs from the mostly gang-related violence discussed up until now, there are two major similarities. First, as in the case of gang-related violence, the ethnic violence in Nigeria primarily involves young men. Second, as in the case of gang-related violence, young men in Nigeria report that being idle, out-of-work and out-of-school are the main reasons they become involved in this violence. The following were the responses of a group of adult men, all Muslim and lower income, regarding the violence:

GB: Why do youth get involved in this violence?

SALIM: Most of the young men involved were dropouts. The elites, they direct them to be violent too.

ALI: Since 1981 I have been involved in every riot there has been. If the violence came, I would be involved. I had no work. I had nothing to do. Why should I not get involved? Three months ago, I became employed as a civil servant. Now that I am getting my daily bread, why should I get involved [in such violence]? Lots of young men do not have this [stable work].

YUSEF: Some of our leaders used this violence to achieve their aims. [*Like what?*] To make their candidates stronger [politicians]. They know that we don't have jobs [and that we'll get involved in this violence].

A group of younger men said similar things:

GB: Why are young men getting involved in these riots?

MOHAMMED: For all these problems, it is the elite who has contributed. They have a political agenda and they motivate youth to participate.

AHEBI: They gave us bad information about what was happening and that is what led to the violence.

OSABE: I heard that because of Sharia, they hired some people to come out against Sharia . . . I don't know if it was a Christian or Muslim who did that. I also heard a rumour that the elites paid young men money to motivate violence.

ALI: Some people believe that to resort to violence is not good. Others believe in using violence, because they are getting something out of it.

This ethnic violence played out in ways that are similar to gang rivalries in the Caribbean, Brazil and the United States. You could be killed by being from the rival group and being in the wrong place at the wrong time:

> They would come up to you on the street and if they were Muslim, they would ask you to recite from the Koran. If they were Christian, they would

ask you to cite from the New Testament. And if you could not, they would kill you like that.

(Mohammed, 29, Kaduna, Nigeria)

Several young men in Nigeria talked about the fear they felt; one young man (now a college student) was initially involved in the riots, but then when he first saw 'blood', he became scared and left:

I was involved [in the violence] in 1987. I was going to an Islamic school, and some people came and told me they [the Christians] were killing Muslims, and can't we retaliate. I was in mosque and they told us that this was a religious war, that this will be a Jihad and that we must go. I was in the adolescent stage, and I thought, 'I am going to Jihad!' But my parents told me not to, so I sneaked out of the house with a friend and we went to an assembly, and I took my grandfather's dagger. And we saw the older men, the fundamentalists, who wanted to propagate the thing. And they told us that the Christians are killing Muslims in this neighbourhood, and most of the youths were aggrieved . . . and annoyed. And then when I saw someone dead, I cried. When I first saw blood, I ran back home . . . And then they started to burn all the churches in our neighbourhood . . . and we went with them [to burn the churches]. We were happy to be there . . . inside a church building holding a stick [to break things inside the church]. And then they started to tell me to steal anything that we could. And then other boys came back from burning and looting another church and told us all they got and all they did, and so we said we can outdo them. So even in civil war, you have young men trying to outdo each other. And then it escalated from one neighbourhood to the whole city.

(Khaled, 27, Kaduna, Nigeria)

This example shows other components of violence, particularly group-related violence. It shows, for example, the adrenaline rush associated with being part of a cause – as in the case of *Jihad!*, which was said with pride and force. It also shows the sense of group belonging, of being caught up with your peers in a single-minded purpose. This young man had other reasons for living and a family what did not support the violence. Too many young men in such settings lack these.

Behind the ethnic components of the violence, there is clear anger over 'elites', adult men, politicians and religious leaders, Christian and Muslim, who are seen as manipulating the situation and benefiting from it. Indeed, in many ways the young men seemed more angry at these 'elites' than they did at rival religious groups or followers of the rival religion. This anger was related to the lack of employment and a clear sense that they were being excluded from the labour market and from the power, opportunities and resources that the older generation – and particularly a few members of the older generation – has. Both Christian and Muslim young men were adamant that the causes of the riots were not merely religious. While they might argue over the meaning of their religions and could get worked up over the implications of Sharia law, they agreed on the fact that religious differences historically existed and did not, in themselves, cause violence:

AHEBI: It is not really a religious crisis . . . I think it is ignorance. If it was a religious issue, we would all fight. It is unemployment.

MOHAMMED: It is a level of understanding between the religions [lack of it]. Why should I fight if I really know what their religion is about? It is the hooligans. It is linked to religion, they [the instigators of the violence] link it, but it is not the cause.

Most journalists writing about this violence have focused on the surface tensions – the clash between Muslim and Christian groups – but deeper tensions are related to access to resources and power. Will Muslims or Christians (and within that, Muslim and Christian men who wield power) rule? For young men, the tensions are often about: How can I get access to a job, to income and to some sense of power, in a place where I feel powerless? This sense of powerlessness among Nigerian young men may even be more prolonged than it is for low-income young men in the United States, Brazil and the Caribbean. Young men in Nigeria remain 'youth' until they are in their thirties. They are 'boys' until they marry, and as such excluded from the status of adulthood. Africa has the highest percentage of its population of any region of the world between the ages of 10 and 24, and the Nigerian young men we spoke with perceived and lived the struggle to find work and opportunities in secondary and higher education. This is the gendered backdrop to their ethnic violence.

Some final reflections on violence

What enables some young men in these settings to stay out of gangs and gang-related violence? For young men in Chicago and Rio de Janeiro, a number of factors are at work, including fear, becoming an involved father, self-reflective abilities, having an alternative identity that provided some status or being part of religious groups (although in Nigeria, being part of certain religious groups was a risk factor). Some of these factors are also relevant for young men in Nigeria who stayed out of riots. Research in other settings reveals similar patterns. When young men in low-income and violent settings find conventional means for attaining identity and status – finishing school; acquiring legal, stable and reasonably well-paid employment; having family members who are able to connect with them; having non-delinquent peers; forming their own family – most young men stay out of gangs.

Non-gang-involved young men in both Chicago and Rio de Janeiro show similar characteristics that seem to explain how is it they stayed out of gangs. These include:

- having a valued, stable relationship or multiple relationships with someone (a parent, a grandparent, a female partner) they would be disappointing if they got involved with the gangs
- having access to alternative identities or some other sense of self that was positively valued by the young man and by those in his social setting, particularly the male peer group but also before young women (for example, being a good student, being a good athlete, having musical skills, having a good job)
- being able to reflect about the risks and costs associated with the violent version of masculinity promoted by gang members
- finding an alternative male peer group that provided positive reinforcement for non-gang-involved male identities.

In later chapters, more of the implications of these findings for working with young men will be discussed.

The example seen of Murilo (at the beginning of this chapter) provides insights on the complexity of male violence. The solutions are not easy; simply providing counselling for Murilo and his parents would not have been enough, nor can we simply blame the social context of a *favela*. We cannot simply associate violence or delinquency with single-parent families, nor the absence of a father, nor merely to low educational attainment. Murilo came from an intact family, had a reasonable educational attainment, and was generally self-reflective. We see in his example a combination of individual factors – an aggressive temperament, probably exacerbated by examples in the home – along with having ties to gang-involved peers.

Finally, what emerges in terms of what factors explain why some young men get involved in gangs or violence and others do not, is a complex inter-action between specific family, peer group and individual characteristics and the greater social context, particularly that of social exclusion. Over-lapping and interacting with these factors are the salient versions of mas-culinities in these communities, in particular a 'hard worker' version of masculinity associated with conventional employment competing with a violent version of masculinity promoted by young men involved in violence. If, however, these two versions of masculinities 'compete' for the loyalties and identities of young men, they also have much in common. Both are identities (overwhelmingly heterosexual) that emphasize men's roles as providers (and the need to have stable income to be recognized as a 'real man'), access to consumer goods and access to women, either as stable or occasional partners or both. Becoming a gang member, and using violence (or risking being a victim of violence), is partly a conscious choice to adhere to an exaggerated – but ultimately traditional – version of manhood.

Aspects of this exaggerated manhood are of course found in the wider local culture in low-income neighbourhoods and beyond – a culture that promotes a man's 'right' to respond to insults to his honour and his right to expect loyalty from female partners, among other things. For example, while gang-related male identities hold sway in *favelas*, their middle-class counterparts have also become visible. In middle-class bars in Rio de Janeiro, groups of middle-class young men (some called 'Pit Boys' after Pit Bulls) have been in the news recently for starting fights with bouncers, with other young men or attacking gays and lesbians at gay bars. Many of these fights have generally been related to altercations over girls, being denied entrance into clubs or bars or disputes between rival peer groups. Indeed, the *comandos* are not the creators of violent versions of masculinity in Brazil, just as gang members in the United States and elsewhere are not. They recreate and sometimes exaggerate these identities from a wider social context that promotes violent and misogynistic versions of manhood.

What is common to both gang-involved and non-gang-involved young men is the fact that they are pressured to achieve the same basic mandates of manhood: to find work, to achieve respect or status and to attract women. What varies tremendously is the means or ways that they go about achieving or attaining this model of adult manhood. Stories of violence, and research on young men's violence are not in short supply, but seldom is this background of manhood included. These examples and stories suggest that the key issue for those young men using violence is that they are seeking to achieve manhood through violent means – they are robbing, killing and dying to live up to a specific, socially reinforced version of manhood.

But there are far more young men, as we have seen, who are seeking to avoid this violent manhood. They are afraid, or they find alternative identities and means to achieve manhood. They have families who can protect them and guide them in appropriate ways, or they have the luck of finding non-violent and pro-social peer groups. In between the headlines and news flashes of violence, these stories of resistance must also be told.

Chapter 6

No place at school

Low-income young men and educational attainment

In most countries, access to good-quality primary and secondary education has been identified as the major policy for improving the well-being and employment prospects of low-income young people. In developing regions, the focus on 'gender' in education has traditionally been on girls. Historically, girls' enrolment has lagged behind that of boys in developing countries (and, a century ago, in northern countries) for a variety of reasons: some cultures thought it was better to preserve the sexual chastity of their daughters by keeping them in the home. In other cultures, girls married and started childbearing early (and in some areas, they still do).

In some settings, girls were seen (and in some places still are) mostly as domestic help and kept in the home to assist with chores. For some low-income families – for whom every child represents a helping hand and for whom income for school fees and supplies are limited – the education of boys is seen as more important than for girls. These realities still exist in some parts of Africa, the Middle East and Asia. Accordingly, international efforts led by UNESCO, the World Bank, the United Nations Children's Fund (UNICEF) and other international organizations have focused on improving formal education enrolment rates for girls.

While major disparities continue in terms of girls' enrolment in some parts of Asia and Africa, these efforts have to a large extent paid off. Girls' enrolment in primary education in developing countries increased from 93 per cent in 1990 to 96 per cent in 1999. According to UNESCO figures for 2002, 86 countries have already achieved gender parity in primary education and 35 are close to doing so (UNESCO 2002). The enrolment rate, of course, is only one indicator of gender equality in schools, and a fairly crude one, but it does give us an indication of gender-related changes that have happened in the school setting. In some school settings, girls are victims of sexual abuse and harassment, so that even if they have access to school, their basic rights are not protected.

As girls' enrolment rates have been increasing, something else has been happening in many countries that achieved gender parity in enrolment rates: the special needs of boys in school started to become evident. In parts of Latin America and the Caribbean, in a few countries in Asia, and in nearly all of Western Europe and North America, girls are completing more years of school than boys and are performing better academically than boys on several measures (reading levels and standardized test scores). Indeed, in some countries in these regions, low-income, urban-based boys are the group most likely to drop out of school and to have the lowest rates of educational attainment. What is going on with low-income boys and young men in school?

In listening to young men, numerous factors emerge. For Anthony, the problem was one of getting drawn into fights:

> I thought about it and I realized it wasn't worth it [getting into fights at school]. It wasn't worth me failing. It wasn't worth [risking] my education and if I keep acting like this [getting in fights] somebody gonna hurt me too. If not I'm gonna end up in jail for hurtin' somebody or I'm gonna get kicked out of school . . . and I'm never gonna make it.
>
> (Anthony, 17, African American, Chicago)

For Tony, in the same high school, staying out of gangs and family stress were part of the equation:

> I been bringing home bad grades and my father said if I keep bringin' home Fs, we gonna have to have a talk about it. I failed History and English and computer class . . . things ain't goin' right [for me]. I'm a Christian but sometimes I think about why am I part of a gang and then I'm a Christian? I wanna know why things don't go right. I miss my Mom [she died a few months before]. That's why things ain't goin' right. I want her back on Earth.
>
> (Tony, 15, African American, Chicago)

Similarly, for Mitch, the problem was staying out of gangs and finding a group of peers who supported him in positive ways:

> I don't make friends [with anybody at school]. I have associates. I would say my best friends are my Mom and God. You can't trust nobody [here at school]. They may be your friend one day and stab you in the back the next . . . You hang out with the wrong crowd [gangbangers] and I woke up one day seeing that tomorrow ain't guaranteed . . . I don't let myself get close to anyone [here at school].
>
> (Mitch, 18, African American, Chicago)

For Salim, a young man in Nigeria, the issue was needing to work: 'I dropped out of school because I wanted to find a faster way to grab money.' For Anderson, in Rio de Janeiro, the problem was a stressed family that had trouble monitoring his behaviour and whereabouts:

When I was little, I didn't have [the chance to study]. Well I guess I did have it, but I wasted it. You know, when you're younger, you don't want to worry about anything, just goofing off. My mother would call me to go to school and I would say that I wasn't going. And I'd take off running because there was no man at the house . . . a man who could run after me and catch me and make me go to school [his father was deceased]. My mother couldn't catch me. Today, now that I'm older, shit, I'm gonna study. Without an education . . . it's already hard [to find a job].

(Anderson, 21, African Brazilian, Rio de Janerio)

Educational attainment and low-income young men

These are not isolated examples. Indeed, secondary school enrolment data during 1998–2000 in Latin America and the Caribbean show that proportionally more girls than boys are enrolled in 21 of 27 countries for which data are available (Pan American Health Organization (PAHO), WHO and Population Reference Bureau (PRB) 2003). The difference ranges from 1 percentage point to 19 percentage points. The English-speaking Caribbean shows some of the largest disparities. As of 1995, public secondary schools in Trinidad and Tobago had about 60 per cent female students and 40 per cent males. Functional literacy tests applied at the end of primary school in Trinidad and Tobago found that between 75 per cent and 89 per cent of girls can read, while only between 56 and 69 per cent of boys are able to do so. When guidance counsellors at public schools in Trinidad and Tobago were asked why they thought boys were faring worse than girls in schools, they focused on one issue: the lack of male role models. They noted that 65 per cent of teachers are women and that male teachers are most likely to be found at the secondary level. This means that most boys reached the age of 10 or 11 never having seen a male teacher. This may be part of the story, but is clearly not all of it (Barker et al. 1995).

Similarly, in Jamaica, as of 2000, 91 per cent of adult women compared to 83 per cent of adult men were literate, and 85 per cent of young women compared to 82 per cent of young men were enrolled in secondary school (UNICEF 2004). At the level of tertiary education, this disparity increases: 68 per cent of students at the University of the West Indies, Mona, Jamaica's largest public university, are female. Various researchers have consistently found that girls in Jamaica, and elsewhere in the English-speaking Caribbean, are more motivated to attend school than boys, or are subject to greater monitoring of their activities and more likely to be encouraged to attend school. Boys in such settings are often either encouraged or allowed to participate to a greater extent in street-based peer group activities, where manhood is often defined as being oppositional to school attendance (Barker et al. 1995).

Similar trends are occurring in some parts of Latin America. Brazil is a case in point. While primary enrolment has now reached nearly 100 per cent in Brazil, a recent analysis of national educational enrolment data found that only 33 per cent of young people aged 15–17 in Brazil are in middle school (*ensino medio*), which would be the appropriate level for their age (O Globo 2002c). Examining educational enrolment data for young people aged 15–24, for Brazil as a whole, 57 per cent of young people in this age range have not completed primary schooling; in the state of Rio de Janeiro, 47.5 per cent of young people 15–24 have not completed primary education (Fernandes 2002).

With respect to gender, there are even greater disparities. Nationwide in Brazil, as of 1996, men had an average of 5.7 years of formal education compared to 6.0 years for women (World Bank 1996). Examining educational data from 1997 for young people aged 10–24, we can see that gender disparities show up starting around age 10 for boys when they begin to leave school at higher rates than girls. For youth ages 15–17, for Brazil as a whole, 43.8 per cent of boys are in school only and 27.8 per cent study and work. For girls in the same age range, 57.5 per cent are only studying and 17.3 per cent work (outside the home) and study. In the same age range, 19.2 per cent of boys only work and do not study, compared to only 8.5 per cent of girls (IBGE 1998). Furthermore, in 1996, 7.9 per cent of young men aged 15–19 were illiterate compared to 4 per cent of young women in the same age range (IBGE 1997).

In a survey of young people in one low-income neighbourhood in Rio de Janeiro, among 218 youth aged 13–19, 20.6 per cent of girls compared to 42 per cent of boys had spent at least one year out of school (they had missed at least one entire year of school) (CESPI (Centro de Estudos e Pesquisas sobre a infância) and Promundo 2001). The same study found that 71 per cent of boys compared to 92 per cent of girls interviewed were currently enrolled in school. Of those boys who had stopped studying, 22 per cent said they left school to work, while more than 30 per cent reported having stopped going to school simply because they '. . . wanted to.' The fact that they were allowed to leave school, or that their families and the school system could not encourage them to attend school, is another indication of the lack of positive social control that could be applied to keep them in school.

Why are boys leaving school?

What is happening then in the public school system for low-income boys and young men? First, it is important to recognize that the public school system in most developing countries and many other parts of the world does not serve well either low-income girls or boys. Throughout the world, school enrolment drops significantly at the secondary level for low-income youth. Too many young people of both sexes are excluded from the school system for reasons that have been well described elsewhere, including:

- early childbearing
- rigid discipline systems that expel any youth who violates school norms
- family stress
- lack of income for school fees
- too few spaces for the number of youth of school-going age
- educational curricula that are irrelevant for the needs of low-income youth
- the need for youth to work to contribute to family income.

Poverty interacts with racial and ethnic-based exclusion as well. In the United States and Brazil, young people of African descent have lower enrolment rates than those of European or Asian descent.

Discussions of boys' difficulties in schools have been limited but are beginning to emerge in Australia, Jamaica, Mongolia, even parts of Africa, and internationally (UNICEF 2004). The traditional argument in some poorer countries has been that boys are more likely to drop out of school early because they are more likely to work outside the home. (Girls work at rates nearly as high as boys, perhaps even higher, when their unpaid domestic work is included.) Indeed, as has been discussed, there are clear social expectations that boys should work outside the home to support themselves and their families, particularly in low-income settings. But more may be going on than the fact that more boys than girls work outside the home.

Various studies suggest that the different ways boys and girls are socialized contributes to the situation. Girls are mostly encouraged to stay in or near the home, while boys are encouraged and urged to spend time away from or outside their homes. Time use studies – in which individuals are asked how they spend their days – confirm that girls are more likely to work in the home or be in the home, while boys are more likely to work outside the home or to be outside the home. In low-income urban settings, girls are more likely to be at home taking care of younger siblings or carrying out domestic chores, while boys are more likely to be hanging out on the streets, playing or working.

Does this socialization in the home for girls encourage positive study habits and staying on task? And is the school environment more conducive to the ways that most girls are socialized in their interaction and ways of learning? Research from Jamaica suggests that boys there are generally socialized to run free while girls are confined to the home. As a result, girls may learn to concentrate on tasks, sit still for longer periods of time and interact with greater ease with female authority figures. Boys on the other hand, may spend more time in unstructured settings, with greater movement and where physical force, rather than concentrating and sitting still, are rewarded. A group of low-income boys in Kingston, Jamaica, interpreted the situation this way:

GB: Why do you think it is that girls are staying school longer than boys?

JOSEPH: They [the boys] hang out with a [male peer] group . . . they see the vibes . . . they hear that school is a stupid thing . . . [the gang of males] pushes weed and cigarette . . . [and they end up liking that more].

GEOFFREY: The girl develops an isolation process [she learns on her own] . . . the girl stays in school because she stays in her room . . . so she learns to like to read.

IAN: It's all in the socialization forces . . . A girl is inside looking at books . . . he the boy, he is outside playing football. The girl just studies.

WILLIAM: The boy and girl have the same brain . . . but the boys says he's better . . . He thinks he doesn't have to study. He thinks it will come naturally to him.

Another major issue for boys in the school system is labelling and stereotyping. Teachers (the majority of whom are women, at least in primary and middle levels) sometimes hold stereotypical images of low-income boys, which may lead them to create self-fulfilling prophecies – they think that boys will be disruptive and drop out of school or be excluded from school and boys in turn are disruptive and leave or are expelled from school (Taylor 1991; Figueroa 1997).

Informal conversations with teachers and observations of the classroom setting suggest that some women teachers may have a difficult time controlling or dealing with the sometimes disruptive and aggressive energy of boys. We saw in Murilo's case examples of parents and teachers overreacting to outbursts or comments that he made. Indeed, in these low-income urban settings, boys spend more time outside the home socializing with predominantly male peer groups whose style of interaction and aggressive energy is probably not conducive to a learning system that requires sitting still for hours at a time. As previously noted, one woman teacher in a public school in Rio de Janeiro pointed ominously to several boys in the classroom setting and told me that she knew they had family members in the *comando*. While she genuinely seemed to want to help the boys in question stay in school, her comments also suggested that some boys are marked or identified as potential troublemakers because of their ties to the *comando*.

Another major factor in boys' school leaving and school troubles is the nature of the male peer group. In many parts of the world, there is a common or normative pattern in which boys between the ages of 10 and 12 feel the need to rebel against rules and often begin 'hanging out' with anti-school peers. In this age range, boys begin to seek greater autonomy. They often perceive that being a 'boy' is to be powerless, and they seek to prove themselves as men. They sometimes chafe at authority and disputes begin over which version of manhood will dominate – recall my personal hippy–kicker experience. For many low-income boys, who see the school-leaving paths of their older brothers, fathers and peers, school is made out to be uncool. A young man in Jamaica said that it was 'uncool' to be seen as a 'head-boy' (a boy who does well in school) among their male peer group.

Researchers in the Caribbean have suggested that for many boys, school is seen as childish; to become a man you must affirm yourself in the outside world, in spaces outside female control (Chevannes 2001). In the case of Trinidad and Tobago, guidance counsellors from public schools suggested that this situation is exacerbated by the fact that there are few male teachers. In these settings, boys may reason: *If this were serious work, men would be involved in teaching.* For many young men, the school thus becomes another home-like environment – dominated by women and girls. Indeed some boys seem to react to the 'feminine' style of the public education setting, seeing it as one more space where – like the home – they feel the need to break free from the control of women. The developmental psychologist Erik Erikson wrote about this phenomenon in the 1960s in the United States and his observations still ring true in some of the settings discussed here:

> The fact that the majority of teachers in our elementary schools are women must be considered here in passing, because it can lead to a conflict with the nonintellectual boy's masculine identification, as if knowledge were feminine, action masculine.
>
> (Erikson 1968: 125)

For some low-income African American boys in the United States, as noted by several authors, succeeding in school sometimes means acting in ways that are seen as 'white' – using a different kind of language, dress and styles of inter-action that are more Anglo-European than African American. In a context of racism and unequal opportunities, to be seen as 'playing white' by your black peers is to be criticized, if not outright ostracized by the peer group.

It is unfortunate but true that it is relatively rare for a low-income, young, urban-based black man to succeed in secondary school. To succeed in school and follow an academic path means that you set yourself apart from the crowd, and in effect chart territories that your peers (and family members) often have not. In such settings, male peers will try to convince you that playing football, baseball or cricket or just hanging out are more interesting than attending school, where you have a rigid schedule and someone – usually a woman, and often a woman from a different social class to yours – who tells you what to do.

In many low-income settings in poorer countries, families and school systems seem powerless to keep low-income boys in school. In the overcrowded, public educational systems in such settings, the educational system often seems content to let young men be expelled: after all, there are not enough slots to go around. In observations in some of the settings described here, only when families were extremely vigilant were they able to counter the indifference of the school system and the anti-school male peer group and keep their sons in school. For example, as we saw previously with Anderson from a *favela* in Rio de Janeiro, there was no adult who was able to help channel his energy into the school system. His mother and grandmother were older and had health problems, and there was no other family member around to gently, but with authority, help Anderson think about this future and his options. He spent several years hanging out on the streets, then selling drugs as part of a *comando*, until he perceived that his life was in danger. When he began to participate in a youth leadership programme we offered, he was able to enrol in night classes and return to school; at the age of 18, he re-enrolled in the third grade (third year of primary school).

Other young men show similar family stresses – factors that contribute to the dropout of boys and girls. For example, several boys in Rio de Janeiro missed a year from school because of a minor illness, because a family member was not able to obtain the right document, or because they skipped class frequently. Only when families were vigilant were they able to reverse this situation.

Traditional and rigid education systems, particularly systems that focus more on maintaining order than engaging students in meaningful ways, reinforce these patterns. For example, the educational system in the English-speaking Caribbean emphasizes the common entrance exam for secondary school, and to enter the best secondary school possible. Young people who do not pass the entrance exam generally enter a post-secondary school, which is essentially a dead end, for the final three years of schooling. They then leave school around the age of 15 or 16 or earlier. Those young people who do not pass the common entrance exams are grouped together with other low-achieving students and in effect labelled as academic failures. Even though they are still in school, they have been marked as being non-academic.

In a group discussion in the Caribbean island of St Vincent with young people – about two-thirds male and one-third female – who had not passed the common entrance exam, they showed anger and frustration and had few expectations that the time they were spending in the classroom would result in anything positive. They were frustrated, and their teachers – who thought their main task was simply to keep the young people occupied – were also visibly stressed. This was a classroom going nowhere and everyone knew it. The young people seemed annoyed at questions about the situation; it was after all asking them to talk about the obvious, dead-end nature of their classroom. A group of researchers had been called to ask young men about their problems in school – and they were clearly labelled as the problems.

That these 'failed' students sat passively in the classroom was a function of the degree of social control that still exists in small islands like St Vincent. There should be little doubt that, assuming things stayed the same, these young men would be out on the streets doing odd jobs, hanging out at the docks or smoking or selling marijuana where most of their peers were, and the girls in the classroom would likely start childbearing soon. Some may see these behaviours as antisocial, but discussions with young men suggest that they are part of a positive defence mechanism to seek out the male group for support when they perceive that the school system and their family do not or cannot assist them.

In Chicago, similar dynamics can be observed – of rigid discipline, of girls performing better than boys and of labelling and stereotyping. The US public education system has a mandate to keep children in school up until the age of 16, and mostly achieves this, even if those children are behind in school, failing or likely will not receive a diploma for completing secondary school. Accordingly, the system mostly operates to keep children in school, but with rigid discipline. The focus is on maintaining order: you may not go anywhere academically, the school tells them, but while you are here you will behave.

In the case of Chicago, it is possible to observe differential treatment by women teachers toward girls. Boys were punished more severely for outbursts. Boys perceived this, and complained about it. Said one African American boy (aged 12): 'Girls get away with everything at school. If they talk back [nothing happens to them] . . . a teacher believes everything a girl say no matter what she say.' Some of the boys, for example, complained that if they used any physical violence against girls, they would be severely punished. Girls, on the other hand, they said, could hit them and nothing would happen.

There were other issues at play that heightened the tensions for boys in schools in low-income areas in Chicago. Starting in the mid-1990s in the United States, there has been a heightened attention to sexual harassment, both between adults in the workplace as well as among students in the school setting. Boys and girls were both aware of the messages in the air about this. While some of these messages were even-handed, others cast boys and men as potential sexual predators. Some boys suggested that girls were using a heightened policing of sexual harassment to their advantage. At one point in a middle school in a mixed Hispanic and African American school, a girl in the hall (probably 12–13 years old) sneered and then yelled 'rape' when a boy her age passed by her. He had done nothing to her, but when she yelled 'rape', other students turned to look and the boy hung his head and tried to act as if she was not talking about him. This boy may have acted differently toward her in other moments; she may in fact have been the victim of attempted unwanted, sexual advances by him or other boys. But in this particular moment, she used the word 'rape' to stigmatize the boy and, by her smile and his reaction, was using it unfairly.

A year in the life of a public school on the South Side of Chicago

Over the course of most of a school year in 1999, I spent one afternoon a week hanging out with a group of young men in a public high school on the South Side of Chicago in a predominantly African American neighbourhood.[1] The neighbourhood where the high school was located was home to a major public housing complex. Some of these housing complexes were being torn down in the 1990s to build smaller residential complexes. Federal public housing planners in the United States had concluded that concentrating the poorest of the poor in large residential facilities led to despair and degradation rather than to hope and improvement.

The high school had all African American students and most of the teachers were also African American. The school had divided itself into small schools within a school – an arts programme, a communication programme, a health professions programme and the like – in an attempt to make students feel more connected, and less as if they were part of a large, anonymous school setting. There were nine 'small schools' within the school, which had a total of about 1500 students. Making these 1500 students feel 'connected' was a daunting objective. Public housing officials had figured out that concentrating the most disadvantaged families in one place did not work; the public education system in Chicago, however, continued to use and build enormous public high schools grouped mostly along income lines.[2]

In 1999, the school was under 'reconstitution,' meaning that its students were not achieving at a high enough level on standardized exams and the city school district was directly managing it. More girls than boys were enrolled at the upper levels, and girls were disproportionately represented among the best-performing students. To give one example, in 1999, 28 students out of about 1500 students at the school had grade point averages which qualified them to be part of the National Honor Society; only 3 were boys.

I interacted mostly with a group of young men involved in a discussion and support group developed by the school's health educator to discuss issues related to sexuality, male–female relationships and HIV/AIDS. In practice, the discussions revolved around all the major issues of these young men's lives. It was run by a young male psychologist, whom we will call Samuel Jones, who was a former star high school basketball player, which gave him some rapport with the young men.

Among the 20 young men in the group, there was Anthony, one of the three male members of the Honor Society, a star football player, and a self-proclaimed Christian. There was Tony, a sophomore, who was trying to stay out of gangs and struggling with his mother's recent death. There was Charlie B, who was into rap and was trying to start his own record label. There was Mitch, a senior, who was trying his best to stay out of gangs, but having trouble doing so. His older brother was in a gang and most of his closest friends were as well. Mitch was a talented football player and struggling to finish high school and trying to get a scholarship to a university on the East Coast. He had attempted suicide once during the year by taking an overdose of pain medication, and was on 'suicide watch', meaning that teachers were asked to watch for danger signs that might signal a pending suicide attempt.

Mr Jones said there were three kinds of young men in the school:

- *Gang members*, also called *Eduardos*. Mr Jones estimated that 10–20 per cent of young men in the school had some tie to gangs, the majority, he says, to 'stay safe . . . and because they feared they would be recruited.' Staying out of gangs was a major challenge for some of the young men; for others it was merely a nuisance.
- *Romeos*, or young men who are after sexual conquests. Mr Jones said of them: 'The Romeo, he's too busy for me [for participating in the guys' group]. He's chasing girls all the time . . . He respects me, but he wants his trophies [his sexual conquests].'
- *The Neutrons*, young men not involved in gangs and not trying to be *Romeos*. These are young men who are, as Mr Jones said: 'trying to do right but . . . people are pulling at him to do other things'.

Mr Jones had an easy-going style that engaged the young men at their level, but he also challenged their behaviour. He intervened when one of them got in trouble for speaking back to a teacher, or when one was going to be cut from the football team because his grades were not good enough. He did not try to get the young men off the hook, but rather sought to challenge their behaviour without alienating them. He also assisted them with their intimate relationships, giving them advice on 'how do deal with the ladies . . . how to treat them right.' The group had a strong message about abstinence and safer sex, and above all, avoiding getting a girl pregnant.

In the school's official and unofficial discourse – like that in the United States as a whole from the late 1990s to 2004 – early childbearing or teenage pregnancy had become the defined evil and problem; it was the reason African American youth were dropping out of school. Whether it was the reason they were dropping out of school is unclear, but it was a reason that many were excluded from school. The school's principal had stated publicly that he did not like teen mothers; when a girl got pregnant, he typically transferred her to another school, if in fact she did not decide (or feel pressured) to drop out altogether.

There were individual classroom and school-wide sessions on sexual abstinence. In one of these sessions, most young people slouched in their chairs and stared at a blank piece of paper in front of them. They were given the task of writing a letter to a peer urging that peer not to have sex and giving them at least three reasons to say no to sex. The teacher showed as little enthusiasm for the task as the students did; she was mandated to teach it, and they were mandated to sit through it.[3] A subtle message from some teachers was that they must save young African American men in particular from their sexual desires and violent instincts.

While students at the school were enjoined to feel proud about their African American heritage and encouraged to 'set your sights high', the focus was on maintaining order. Police were stationed at the front door of the school, where students passed through a metal detector to come in. Some of the young men told of being harassed by police. The discipline system gave points off for certain behaviours. Forms were filled out with discipline complaints and a discipline department meted out punishment, called parents and monitored students in detention.

Expulsion was widely used as a method of discipline. The young men were clearly aware of these messages and of the principal's expressed 'zero tolerance' policy toward misbehaving. One young man said: '[we all know we have to watch ourselves] . . . 'cause we all know that the principal . . . he has gotten rid of the students that he know is not gonna do well in school . . . and I would say it has its positive points from that'.

Sitting in a classroom session, it is possible to observe these dual, sometimes confusing messages, of praise and threats. One teacher (a woman) told her classroom: 'You are the cream of the crop. You have the right to feel good about that.' Later in the same session, the teacher told them: 'I'm going to kick your butt because society is going to.' This was education focused on keeping order, with the message that young African Americans must learn to have structure in their unstructured lives. There were, of course, notable teachers, many clearly dedicated to their jobs, but keeping order took up considerable classroom time and energy.

All of the young men in the group stayed in school during the 1999 academic year – this in a setting where about one in four boys dropped out every year. In spite of pregnancy scares, a suicide attempt, problems with grades, getting in trouble (for speaking back to a teacher or skipping class) and pressures to join gangs, the young men in the group all stayed in school. In interviews with the young men, it became clear how important it was to have a small-group space where they connected with someone who understood and accepted them, and with whom they could identify. For most of the young men, Mr Jones was the first adult who treated them as if they were special and as if they and their time were important. Said one of the young men:

> Mr Jones is that type of person where you can talk to. He like a father fig-
> ure . . . Mr Jones put like everyone up under his wings. I don't think that it's
> one person in this school that don't like Mr Jones. Mr Jones is like a cool
> person. Every since then, every time class started he used to say: 'First of all
> I like to thank you for your time' [imitating Mr Jones' gestures] and after that
> people will be like he is just a cool person.
>
> (Lamar 17, African American, Chicago)

For many of the young men, it was the first time they interacted with an adult who treated them as if their time, ideas and energy were important.

It would be unfair and untrue to conclude that girls fared well in this set-ting. But there are certain gender-specific challenges that boys faced. One was the attitude of teachers that as young African American men, they were both oversexed and potentially violent. The discipline system and all its bureaucracy as described here, was mostly developed to control the behav-iour of boys. Boys were overrepresented in detention, in expulsions and in discipline problems in general. The police and metal detectors were focused mostly on young men, trying to keep male violence out of the school. Gangs recruited them, trying to draw them into violence.

For a young, black man to succeed in this school setting was to stand out from his peers; witness the handful of boys in the Honor Society. To be vis-ible like this, to be seen as succeeding academically, brought with it the risk that his peers would reject him. To move ahead of one's peers academically was to be seen as snobby and to risk social isolation. Some of the boys did succeed; several graduated and a few went on to university.

What emerges from this example, is that it is possible to revert the school-related challenges that low-income young men face. A group of young men in a setting where many young men drop out of school, if supported by car-ing and committed professionals – like Mr Jones – can reasonably succeed in school. What is disturbing is that the system is content to support just a handful of young men; indeed the system seems designed so that only a few will 'make it'. There were about 20 young men in Mr Jones' group, but there were at least 700 young men in the high school. If programmes like this work to keep young men enrolled in school, an obvious question emerges: what about the other 680?

Does school bring income for low-income young men?

Another relevant question in examining young men's school woes is whether schooling is worth it in terms of greater earnings or employment opportunities for low-income boys. Do low-income young men perceive that schooling provides a return on the investment? Does it in fact increase the income and employment prospects for young men? One of the reasons that low-income young men are dropping out of school in the Caribbean, according to some researchers, is that they have seen that having a university education or completing secondary school does not necessarily bring greater job options. The small island economies in which they live are favouring a mostly female service and information technology industry. Low-income men are likely to work in low-paying, agricultural-based work, as day labourers or as delivery persons and the like. For most of these jobs, it is not necessary to finish secondary education.

Furthermore, an analysis of data from Brazil confirms the fact that educational attainment for socially marginal young people does not lead as directly to higher income as it does for middle-class youth. In 2002 a study commissioned by the International Labour Organization compared average earnings by years of schooling for greater metropolitan Rio de Janeiro as a whole and for low-income areas (Souza and Urani 2002). This analysis shows that for greater Rio de Janeiro as a whole, the average income with just four years of schooling is nearly equal to the average earnings for those with 11 years of education from low-income areas in the city. In addition, among low-income residents who reach university-level education, average income is less than half of the average earnings for a person with university-level education for the city as a whole.

What these data imply is that marginalization for low-income youth is more that just a lack of access to education. Class, race and gender barriers, along with more limited social capital, mean that some young men report and perceive that education has little measurable impact on their employment status and earnings, or in any case, less impact than for middle-class youth. In low-income, urban settings such as these, it becomes even more difficult to motivate a low-income young man to stay in school. Furthermore, it may be that being in school provides relatively little status or identity for a young man, compared to working or being in a gang.

Research from the Caribbean confirms similar tendencies. A study on school-leaving youth in Jamaica (Trevor Hamilton and Associates, 1995) concluded that for some low-income young men, leaving school was a rational decision, given that it had little impact on social mobility. The same inquiry also confirmed that a secondary education in Jamaica is no guarantee of employment. Among 1200 youth leaving secondary school, the researchers found that of those who entered the labour market full-time, 53.6 per cent were unemployed one year after completing school. Youth unemployment is approximately 40 per cent of young people aged 15–24 in Jamaica. For males at lower educational levels, unemployment is lower than it is for females, suggesting that males who drop out of school are generally able to find some kind of employment, much of it in the informal sector or of a makeshift kind (cited in Barker et al. 1995).

Clearly, educational attainment does contribute to higher income, as numerous analyses have confirmed. However, this association is not evenly experienced. Thousands of youth, particularly low-income young men, are aware that the odds are stacked against them in the educational system, and that in any case a secondary education is no guarantee of employment. Others come from families and live in situations where they are unable to stay in school, or are expelled from school, even when they and their families know this will harm them in the long run. Few 10–13-year-olds have a long-term horizon; they are interested in fitting in for the short term and getting through a day in school without fighting. For those of us from middle-class families, our parents and teachers generally keep us focused on the long run. Indeed, virtually all children need support and guidance to be convinced that school is worth it. However, too few parents in low-income settings are able to provide this guidance, particularly with the power of anti-school male peer groups.

Thus, too many young men follow the academic path of Bob Marley, who dropped out of school to the chagrin of his mother to pursue his music career. As the following statements from young men in Kingston, Jamaica, attest, the situation has not changed much since Marley's time:

GB: What is it like for a young man to find work these days?

THOMAS: Young boys . . . think they can be a DJ [dub-rap singer] – they think there's a lot of money in it . . . so he thinks 'I can be a DJ' . . . so he drops out of school. Most of them can't even write the words they sing.

PETER: It is very difficult to find a job these days . . . you have to have lots of subjects . . . you have to have contacts.

ANDY: You can pass secondary with five subjects and still not find a good job.

Engaging boys in school

Schools in low-income urban settings should see themselves as being in a marketplace of competing versions of manhood. They are in fact competing for the hearts and minds of young men. In some settings, the competition is quite obvious: anti-school peer groups or gangs. Indeed, as a contrast to the style of passive learning that often characterizes public schooling in the region, it is useful to look again at what it means to be in a gang. Being in a gang implies action, alacrity, tuning in and maintaining a state of alertness (Souza and Urani 2002). These are all traits that may be keenly suited to the way boys are socialized outside the home. Of course, other activities, like conventional work, being part of a musical group or participation in a football team may also be interesting and engaging to boys for the same reasons – they imply action and require tuning in and maintaining alertness. The point is that the public education system in these settings, particularly in lower-income areas, probably provides few spaces or opportunities for boys to feel engaged in these same ways (and girls for that matter).

Mihaly Csikszentmihalyi (2002) introduced the concept of 'flow' to refer to a state of optimal concentration when creativity combined with total involvement seems to consume us to an extent that nothing else seems to matter. For most individuals, 'flow' is achieved in activities that are self-selected or at least involve some degree of personal selection or control. Individuals report 'flow' experiences in sports activities, in meaningful workplaces, and in school settings where their desires and experiences are taken into account and their energy is focused. Young men involved in gang activities or ethnic violence – focused on a common enemy and experiencing an adrenaline rush – probably experience something like flow. Boys frequently experience the sensation of flow in some sports activities. However, few school settings – or youth programmes in general – seem to be successful in creating this kind of optimal and pleasurable engagement.

There has been some initial programme development related to the special challenges that low-income boys face in the United Kingdom, Australia, Canada, limited parts of the Caribbean and the United States. The challenge with such initiatives is to avoid reinforcing gender stereotypes by suggesting, for example, that all boys learn one way and all girls in a different way. Many boys are faring well in school, and seem to adjust to it well, just as there are girls who do poorly. In examining these gender differences, we should keep in mind that individual differences and class differences are equally or more important than aggregate gender differences. Nonetheless, there is a need for special attention to boys' realities in public education in many parts of the world, particularly low-income boys. The response should be to consider the ways that gender socialization can create specific challenges for girls and boys. Girls, for example, often drop out for reasons related to unplanned pregnancies, while boys drop out for some of the reasons we have previously cited. The point is: both boys and girls in low-income settings too often drop out of school or are pushed out of school for reasons that interact with or are directly related to gender.

If not school, where?

A strong tendency in youth and education policy in many countries has been toward the universalization of school (involving all youth) and an integrated school day (involving youth all day long). But it is clear that, for many low-income boys, school is not the place where most of their socialization takes place. The problem is that like the school, there are relatively few structured community-based programmes (after-school programmes, youth centres, health posts, etc.) that openly accept and welcome low-income young men.

In a study in Brazil, in low-income neighbourhoods, boys were slightly more likely than girls to participate in some activity outside the home – whether recreational, cultural or religious (CESPI/USU – Universidade Santa Ursula and Instituto Promundo 2001). However, boys were more likely to participate in unstructured or informal groups – a skateboarders group, an informal football group, a group of graffiti-painters, and the like. Girls, when involved in social groups, were more likely to be involved in organized youth groups, whether recreational, cultural or religious. In these organized or structured groups, it is more likely that adults are present and there is more supervision of the activities. Such trends have also been observed in other settings.[4]

The age-old question is whether low-income young men do not like to participate in formal or structured youth groups, or if it is the case that few structured groups exist that invite them. The answer is probably both. In many of the settings described here, for example, there are few structured youth programmes that welcome them, but this varies by neighbourhood. In the case of the English-speaking Caribbean, debates have gone on since the 1940s about what to do about 'rude boys' (the term for low-income, urban-based young men). Researchers conclude that in many cases, low-income youth – and young men in particular – do not take advantage of programmes, even when they exist. The chief reason is that they no longer have faith in the system. In addition, few of these programmes engage young people in optimal, creative and meaningful ways that resemble 'flow'. Others find that structured youth programmes seem too much like school. As one member of staff at a youth programme in Jamaica said: 'The drug "dons" [traffickers] promote themselves to the youth. We have to promote our programmes too if we are to get the youth's attention.' In talking with young men in various parts of the English-speaking Caribbean, many perceived that involvement in drug pushing, drug cultivating or gangs resolved many immediate needs, particularly financial pressures and the desire for status – and acquiring a visible male identity.

These attitudes of low-income young men in the Caribbean, Latin America and Africa – who want money in their pocket today to maintain a lifestyle based in part on images they receive from Europe and North America – must be considered when elaborating new programmes to meet their needs. Low rates of school enrolment and low participation in structured youth programmes mean that large percentages of young men do not regularly interact with or have contact with any structured, social environments. Given that many urban-based, low-income young men in these settings come from single-parent households or from households where both parents have to work – sometimes up to two jobs – this means that many young men have little supervision and attention. Too many of these young men have no place at school, and no place in reasonably structured settings where they can be themselves while also being challenged and engaged in positive ways.

We have seen some examples of how to redress these issues. Special support groups of the kind run by Mr Jones in Chicago are one of those; the challenge is how to scale them up to reach more young men. Remedial educational opportunities, including night school, and accelerated diploma programmes can also sometimes be useful. Tying formal education to vocational training is another example. Finally, teachers and parents must be engaged in the process, reflecting about their expectations, their challenges, their stereotypes – and ultimately working with young people and their families to forge solutions.

Chapter 7

'If you don't work, you have to steal'

Low-income young men and employment

ANDERSON: [Work isn't] everything, but almost everything.

GB: What does it mean [for a man] to work?

MURILO: You have to work. Because you want to have your [own] things and at least when you're 20 or 25, you want your things organized . . . together [have a family and support yourself]. And if you don't work, you're have to steal to make a living. You're not going to be [as a man], walking around with nothing to do or wear. I prefer to work [rather than steal].

Work and producing income are the key requisites for being a man in most cultures. Where work is hard to come by and becoming socially recognized as a worker is difficult, these issues become accentuated. The present generation of young men is part of the largest generation or cohort of young people that the world has ever seen (both proportionally and in absolute numbers). When young people line up for a job interview or to take a civil service exam, there are more other young people competing with them for these same jobs than ever before.

To take a concrete example, in 2003, the city of Rio de Janeiro announced that it was accepting applications for an additional 600 sanitation workers, a position with a monthly salary of about US$250, including benefits. The requisites were having completed primary school and being at least 18 years of age. More than 20,000 men – mostly in their twenties – lined up with their applications. The police had to be called in to maintain order and control fights and scuffles that ensued. For most people, this 'youth boom' is a figure on a chart or graph – a bulge in the population pyramid. For young men lining up for relatively low-paid sanitation jobs, the 'youth boom' is the very real fact of there being 19,999 other young men trying to get the same job as you (O Globo 2003).

There are examples like this elsewhere. In Nigeria, men in their late thirties said they had spent more than five years trying to get low-level civil service jobs. One of them said: 'To get one of these jobs, you have to bribe someone or know someone. You have to pay 45,000 *naira* [about US$375] just to get your application in. Even that money does not guarantee that you will get the job.' US$375 represented about three to four months' wages for these low-income men, but they said that there was no shortage of men and women willing to pay this bribe.

It comes then as no surprise that employment – acquiring work and income – weighs heavily and constantly on the minds of low-income men. In group discussions on issues such as HIV/AIDS, violence prevention or violence against women, the topic of conversation returns to employment: 'What we really want is work.' As Anderson put it, for a man 'work is almost everything.' This chapter will examine some of the recent trends in greater detail and reflect further about the challenges that low-income young men face in terms of acquiring employment.

It must be recognized from the start that the employment situation of young women is also difficult. For many, paid employment comes in addition to tremendous responsibilities and work in the home, which may include child care for those who are mothers. Furthermore, sexual harassment and abuse are too commonplace for working women. Young men interviewed in Nigeria reported that young women seeking civil service jobs are frequently forced to exchange sexual favours to move their application up or to advance professionally. The massive entrance of women into the workforce – which happened in northern countries starting from the 1950s onward, in the 1970s and 1980s in Latin America and more recently in some other southern countries – has been the driving force behind changes in gender norms. In many countries, women historically contributed to household income and household production, including agricultural production, but such contributions were not valued (and still are not). This emphasizes how young men's participation in the workplace cannot be discussed without also recognizing the dynamics of women's roles in the workplace.

Any jobs out there?

As mentioned in Chapter 4, data from the International Labour Organization suggest that as many as 70 million young people aged 15–24 are currently unemployed, and that in the next 10 years, 500 million young people will enter the world's workforce. While rates vary by country, by urban–rural settings and by educational attainment, data confirm that youth employment is two to three times higher than adult unemployment in most developing countries. In sub-Saharan Africa, only one-quarter of young people (aged 15–24) are economically active; given the extent of poverty in Africa, we can assume that many more young people would like to be employed but cannot find work (Okojie 2003). In many countries in Asia-Pacific, youth unemployment makes up over 30 per cent of total unemployment (Ghee 2002). In Latin America and the Caribbean, young people account for more than 50 per cent of unemployed workers (Hopenhayn 2002). These figures use official definitions of unemployment, referring to individuals who are actively seeking work, but cannot find it. Left out of this definition is underemployment, referring to those adults and young people in positions that pay miserably, offer no advancement or too few hours.

There are also gender-specific trends in the workplace in many countries. In Latin America and the Caribbean, women's participation in the labour market has increased since the early 1980s, while men's has either declined or remained about the same (United Nations 1995, cited in Engle 1997). These trends have led to shifts in arrangements for child care and have called into question men's generally limited involvement in domestic tasks, including child care. In much of the region, men and women in lower-income groups face economic instability and declining wages, and some men and women are working longer hours in jobs with less stability even when they can find stable work.

While some young men say that women are faring better than they are, we must be cautious about making broad generalizations. For example, an analysis of employment and income trends among men in Argentina, Brazil and Costa Rica from 1988 to 1997 found that some groups of men faced declining income, but not all men, and not even all men in the lowest income groups (Arias 2001).[1]

One of the responses of families to men's uncertain employment, and the search for employment, is migration. In South Africa, Central America, Mexico and the Caribbean, male migration is partly the explanation for high rates of female-headed households. In Honduras, for example, in 2001, an estimated 600,000 persons were working outside the country (representing more than 10 per cent of the country's total population), 75 per cent of whom were men. Their income remittances are said to represent up to one-quarter of the Honduran gross national product (Alatorre 2002).

If trends regarding men's employment are uneven and vary by country, what is clear is that work is a central component – if not *the* central component – of men's identities. While considerations of men and their work have often focused on the impact of income on family well-being, employment and income have other meanings, too. Work gives men their main social identities and provides them with their chief socially recognized function. Women and children generally view fathers in these ways as well. In a sample of rural-based children in Peru, 50 per cent said that their father's principal role was to work, followed by 20 per cent who said their principal role was to buy them things (also related to work), followed lastly by 13 per cent who said it was to help in the home (Garcia-Hjarles 2001).

Catching the big, big black fish: young men and work in the Caribbean

In 1995, as part of a UN study on young men and involvement in drug production and trafficking, interviews were carried out with young men on four islands in the English-speaking Caribbean. Respondents reported without hesitation that the reason for involvement by young men in drug trafficking was the lack of stable and meaningful employment. While statistics on youth unemployment are not always available nor uniform, in Jamaica, more than 40 per cent of young people aged 15–24 are unemployed, as are 49 per cent of young people aged 15–25 in Trinidad and Tobago. One only has to walk around Jamaica's garrison communities (called 'garrison' because of the degree of control by organized gangs, called posses), or the dock areas in St Vincent, to see the number of young men, who are, as Caribbeans say, limin' – hanging out with no place to go and nothing to do.

On the island of St Vincent, young men represent about 20 per cent of arrests on drug-related charges. Every year, several hundred young men enter the prison system or the one government-funded residential mental health facility. Those who used drugs as well as sold them generally received a 'lighter' sentence and were sent to the mental institution. On a visit to this facility (as noted in Chapter 4), nurses were observed dispensing psychotropic medication to patients whose only 'mental illness' seemed to be marijuana use. In short, the prison system and the mental health system in St Vincent mostly receive low-income and out-of-work young men.

Government officials cited growing cultivation of marijuana in the hard-to-reach volcanic hills in St Vincent, and there was evidence that a large number of out-of-school youth were participating in the cultivation and selling of marijuana. Bananas were the chief cash crop on the island, but their price fluctuated significantly and often depended on the status of trade agreements and tariffs in the European Union and United States. Said one out-of-school young man: 'Farming goes up and down. Right now the price is down. *Ganja* [marijuana] means easier, quicker money . . . When the soil can't grow bananas, you grow *ganja* . . . You have to do something.'

In one of the coastal villages, young men cited banana farming and fishing as the only livelihood options available. When asked what they fished for, they answered (in the sing-song style of Caribbean pidgin English, which often repeats adjectives for emphasis): 'Big, big black fish . . . up to 30, 40 feet long.' Would that be a whale? 'Yup, 'em a whale.'

The place they lived was a former whaling village. While whaling was uncertain, it nonetheless offered stable employment, with young men joining in as informal apprentices. There was a clear identity for men and social meaning given to capturing a 30-foot pilot whale – a big, big black fish – which was a much-celebrated event. The big, big black fish provided food and various raw materials to feed and maintain several families.

Men who once captured whales were now having to migrate for work, leaving their families behind. Others were trying to make a living selling bananas or other crops, facing the unstable prices of the market. Some young men (and adult men) turned to drug cultivation. The rolling and often inaccessible hills of St Vincent are ideal for growing marijuana. Said one young man: '[There are many young people involved in selling drugs] because you make enough money to buy a house in a week. If you work a regular job, you will need to work for years.'

If they are not working, what are young men doing? The English-speaking Caribbean illustrates the trend of too many young men with no place to go and nothing to do. The National Skills Training Programme (the government vocational training programme for youth) estimates that 3000 young people in St Vincent take the common entrance exam every year, of which one-half pass, leaving an estimated 1500 youth excluded from secondary school, disproportionately males. Out-of-school young people in St Vincent who are motivated to seek services such as vocational training sometimes find these services; however, there is a large population of out-of-school young people who lack the motivation to seek such services and only a limited number of spaces. Some young people said that existing programmes for them were 'boring', 'just talk' or served no purpose.

This situation leaves a large population of marginalized youth, the majority males, who spend time looking for short-term work, but mainly just limin'. The majority continue to live at home (often in a single-mother household), while some may leave to live with a group of friends in an abandoned house in a low-income district.

Similar trends can be found elsewhere. In Jamaica, there are an estimated 150,000 out-of-school youth, just hanging out or working in the informal sector – if working at all. This pattern repeats in Nigeria, the United States and Brazil: large cohorts of young men out of work and out of school, and too many young people seeking too few places in vocational training programmes.

Brazil offers a useful example. Unemployment rates in low-income communities in Rio de Janeiro are around 12.4 per cent, compared to a national average of 7.3 per cent and an overall citywide rate of 5.2 per cent. As previously cited in Chapter 5, household per capita earnings are R$134 (about US$48) in low income neighbourhoods compared to a city average of about R$700 (about US$250) (Souza and Urani 2002). Since the early 1990s, there has also been an increase in occupation in the informal sector among young people aged 18–24 and other age groups as well in Brazil.[2]

In addition, due in part to increasing (but still low) educational enrolment and to efforts to reduce and eradicate child labour in Brazil, there has been a declining participation of young people aged 15–17 in the labour market. At the same time, there has been an increase in unemployment among those aged 18–24, whose unemployment rates are about twice the national unemployment rates (Souza and Urani 2002). Specifically, data from 1991 to 2000 show a decrease in the number of youth aged 15–17 working, from about 30 per cent to just under 15 per cent for boys and from less than 20 per cent of girls to fewer than 10 per cent of girls working for the Rio de Janeiro metropolitan area as a whole. Nonetheless, in low-income areas of Rio de Janeiro, the proportion of young people aged 15–17 who work continues to be high, nearly double the workforce participation rates for the city as a whole. In some low-income areas, nearly 50 per cent of young people aged 15–17 work, with higher rates for boys (Souza and Urani 2002).

As previously mentioned, young men are far more likely to be working outside the home than young women. For youth aged 15–19 in Brazil as a whole, as of 1999, 42 per cent of young women were working (outside the home) compared to 61 per cent of young men. For the 20–24 age range, 64 per cent of young woman were working in 1999 (up from 56 per cent in 1989) compared to 89 per cent of young men (down from 91 per cent in 1989). In short, trends in many developing countries suggest that unemployment is a chronic and growing problem, particularly for young, less-educated workers (Arias 2001).

The meaning of work and the pressure to work

But what does work and the lack of work mean to young men? And what does it mean when young men are denied access to what they most need to achieve socially recognized manhood? As shown earlier, work is necessary for family formation, in order to be able to attract female partners and to form a family. The lack of stable employment in effect traps young men in childhood or adolescence.

Young men are also selective about work; not just any work was sufficient to achieve socially recognized manhood. Odd jobs that require you to sell on the streets, or that offer intermittent income are generally not enough to achieve manhood. Young men who can – that is young men whose parents were working, even in low-income jobs – say they avoid working in situations they find degrading: selling on the streets or on buses, or lining up with dozens of other young men whenever a new construction site opened up. They, like their parents, and the middle class around the world, want reasonably stable employment, the kind that pays benefits and offers a secure income.

Between the ages of 14 and 17, males in lower and lower middle income families in many parts of the world are expected to begin contributing financially to their families and/or providing for themselves. Some young men show visible signs of stress when they talk about the pressure they feel to find a job. Essentially, young men are asked to do something – acquire and maintain employment – that they are generally ill prepared to do and which is extremely difficult to do in the current economic climate. In addition, the risk of not fulfilling this role is to be reminded that one is not a 'true man'. Said a Brazilian young man: 'A guy at 17 or 18 has to worry about getting a job so he can take care of himself. Up until then nothing was forced on him . . . he had no responsibilities.'

Another young man in Rio de Janeiro said he would do everything he could to ensure that his son did not have to experience the same pressure that he did to work at an early age. He said: 'I feel pressured to work. I'm not going to make my son work [like I had to].'

What happens to a young man's sense of self when he is not able to meet these expectations and find adequate employment? Many young men report examples of fathers who abandoned their families, were physically abusive of their wives and children, turned to alcohol or faced other problems as a result of unemployment or being unable to fulfil their socially designated role of provider. Since most societies define a man's principal role to be the breadwinner, men face considerable stress when they are not able to fulfil that function. For young men in female-headed households, the pressure to find work to substitute for the income of the absent father or adult male provider can be even greater. Said one young man in a mother-headed household in Brazil:

> My mother insists that I find a job. Sometimes I run away from her so I don't have to answer [when she asks me if I found a job]. I look and I look but I can't find a job. It's hard.
>
> (Arturo, 22, African Brazilian, Rio de Janeiro)

Women and mothers in these settings are clearly able to see the stress that young men face. In one group discussion with adult and young women in Rio de Janeiro, one woman said:

> these days looking for work is hard [for a man] . . . he'll look but he won't find anything, and when he finds something it will pay just a little. So then he'll start a family when he's still young. They'll have children right after that [and he has to support them] . . . I mean, I think it's difficult for men. The doors don't open.
>
> (Lucia, 34, African Brazilian, Rio de Janeiro)

Anderson, who was previously introduced, had participated in drug trafficking, in large part because of pressure he felt to contribute financially to his household (in which both his mother and grandmother were unable to work). He said this about the meaning of work:

> [Work isn't] everything, but almost everything. You know [if you work], you'll have some money in your pocket. I mean if you don't have work, you see

men get involved in all kinds of trouble. You want to kill someone with a knife in your hand. I've seen a lot of hard workers get a weapon and start to rob buses just to make ends meet. You need the money. When a guy is working, he's not gonna get rich, but he'll get by. When you have work, you're better off, better for yourself, and nobody wishes you a hard time.

(Anderson, 21, African Brazilian, Rio de Janeiro)

Indeed, young men were keenly aware of the dire actions that some men would resort to when they were out of work. Said one young man:

[When a man is out of work] . . . he's gonna lose control, start to rob, do whatever he can to get money . . . if I go out and try to get a job and I don't find it, and I see that there's all kinds of things we need at home that I can't get . . . then your mind starts to change . . . I mean unemployment is rough. Then the money you get is . . . not enough to make ends meet. Then a guy will start to get desperate. If he's a guy without a head [meaning that he does not think for himself], he's gonna rob, gonna become a gangster.

(Jeferson, 19, African Brazilian, Rio de Janeiro)

Another young man in Rio de Janeiro said:

This guy who lived on my street, they say that they ran out of cooking gas at home. His son was going hungry. So when it's like that, he went out to rob. He's still in jail for that . . . He had a job before that. He was a carpenter, but he couldn't find work . . . he's been in jail for a long time now.

(Anderson, 20, African Brazilian, Rio de Janeiro)

Young men in Nigeria showed similar struggles in finding work. Many described themselves as being stuck as 'youth'. Because they could not acquire employment, they were not recognized as adult men and thus could not get married. In the Nigerian context, a young man is expected to support not only himself and his nuclear family, but also in many cases his extended family.

A group of adult men, all of whom were currently employed in low-level civil service jobs, said they had to pay bribes to secure their jobs. In the volatile Nigerian economy, civil servant jobs – even if they paid poorly – were coveted. When asked what happened to men who did not find this kind of job, they responded:

ALI: . . . they [unemployed men] won't want you to rob, but they want you to do just about anything else to have money for the family.

YUSEF: But if you are a civil servant, your family will be proud of you.

AHMED: If you are a bricklayer [an unstable, low-paying position], you are not happy as a man. You will always be thinking, how will I get money to help my family? If you are a civil servant, you are happy.

MOHAMMED: Most of all, if you are a civil servant, society will recognize you. If you are a casual [itinerant] worker, they will not recognize you.

YUSEF: If you are a civil servant, everyone [your family] relies on you. Even after you are a civil servant, there is pressure, because even more people come to you for help, wanting your money.

Behind the frustration was anger – particularly anger at those older men who controlled access to jobs and wielded power:

ALI: . . . our elders [older men] do not want us to succeed. They want us to be their servants forever . . . they are the ones who make the Muslims and Christians go to the streets and loot houses and shops. They are the ones behind it. They should know that as soon as we have the chance, we will kill them all [he said this with a visible anger on his face].

A group of young, unemployed men in Nigeria, between the ages of 19 and 21, also showed anger toward elites and elders, whom they said only look out for themselves and try to keep the jobs and income to themselves. One of the young men said: 'In our communities, there is plenty of work for us . . . bad work . . . they exploit us and want us to do the hard work like lifting and buildings things.'

In all of these settings, young men said that work is important for being respected in their immediate social group and also outside their communities. As we saw in Chapters 2 and 3, for low-income young men in these settings, venturing into the broader community or into middle-class neighbourhoods brings with it a constant risk of being harassed by police. In Nigeria, the risk was being harassed by military forces or soldiers who were sent to areas of the country where riots had taken place. Thus, having stable work – which might be identified by having a uniform or an identity card – is also coveted for the protection it offered. Police and soldiers respect young men with stable employment. In contrast, they expect that 'idle' and unemployed young men will be troublemakers or 'hooligans', and treat them as such.

As noted earlier, some young men in Nigeria feel unable to become socially recognized adult men because of their lack of employment. Young men in Brazil reacted in a slightly different way. Some young men in Rio de Janeiro are keenly aware of how difficult it is to find work, and thus seek to stay out of the job market for as long as they can. It is, they reason, better to be a 'boy' longer than to be pressured to be a man and not able to achieve manhood by finding work. This is not unlike what many middle-class youth do. The difference is that in the intervening years between childhood and acquiring stable employment, most middle-class youth are continuing their education and thus enhancing their future job prospects.

In many of these settings, military service can be an opportunity for acquiring employment, or at least staying out of the job market for a little longer. Many young men in the Caribbean, Brazil and the United States said they saw the military as a fallback if they could not find work. In the case of Brazil, all men aged 17 are required to register for military service, which used to be universal for young men. However, with the large cohort of youth, the Brazilian military has access to more young men than it needs. Thus, it too has become selective. Only a few young men are invited to serve, and typically those with higher educational attainment. Many young men of conscription age were disappointed when they were not called for military service. Some young men in Chicago were involved in the Reserve Officer Training Corps, a pre-training programme for young men and women who want to pursue military careers. It, too, had become more selective. In situations of scarce employment, the military became an attractive, but elusive, alternative.

No job, no woman, no family

Having work is directly linked to a young man's ability to attract young women and form a family. Parents, potential female partners and parents of potential partners all assess the employment prospects and realities of young men. Said one young African American man in Chicago, with bitterness and anger in his voice: 'Girls only want one thing from you. If you out of work, they don't want you. You can clean the toilet and care for the baby, but if you out of work, she don't want you.'

A group of young and out-of-work men in Nigeria confirmed this pressure and the link between family formation and employment:

ADENIYI: I can't get married now because I can only get married when I have money. The moment I get money, I will get married. I have a girlfriend and I share money with her. Something might come of it, since I have some money . . . but I do not have enough money to get married.

AHBED: I don't think of marriage now, because when I get some money, I want to go back to school . . .

MOHAMMED: I don't get married because I don't have any work. I have a girlfriend but no work.

For a young man, being able to support oneself and one's family financially is generally a precursor to forming a stable relationship and starting childbearing. Clearly, many young men and women have children before they have acquired stable employment. But a young man is more desirable as a partner if he has stable employment, and his participation with children he may have will be directly influenced by whether he is employed. For other young men, having an unplanned child can be an impetus to acquire employment. In any case, it is clear that employment is directly linked to when and under what circumstances young men form stable relationships, father children and the degree of involvement they have with those children.

In the Caribbean, many low-income men start fatherhood within casual relationships in their adolescence, often as a way of affirming manhood. In some countries in the English-speaking Caribbean, the majority of first children are born into what are called 'visiting unions' between young, unmarried partners. In Jamaica, for example, only 16 per cent of women in their childbearing years are married. In the majority of cases, young mothers and their children live with the extended family, or pass children to other members of the extended family to care for. The young fathers usually maintain a visiting, non-resident relationship with their children. Many young fathers migrate for work and spend some time away from their children (Brown and Chevannes 1998).

Many of these fathers support the young mother and child during the child's first year and beyond, but most of these first relationships do not last. Often, these early relationships are discouraged by the girl's family, who hope for better marital prospects later on – which means they want their daughter to find a partner who has a job – or reject the young man for his inability to provide for the mother and child.

As the parents get older, they may move into common-law relationships (often with another partner) and for a smaller number, into formal marriage. Children from these early relationships may join the new family or remain outside of it. Whether fathers maintain regular contact with these 'outside' children (children from previous relationships) depends on many factors, but particularly the relationship between the parents. While childbearing outside of marriage has been criticized by some community leaders as being immoral or dysfunctional, many Caribbean researchers argue that this is a functional and historically based pattern to ensure family survival in the face of post-slavery poverty and lingering social exclusion, particularly the unemployment and underemployment of men (Brown and Chevannes 1998). Indeed, this is one of the clearest examples of how men's participation in families is directly linked to their employment status or job prospects.

Unfortunately, the link between employment and family formation for men has not been adequately discussed. The traditional view in the field of gender studies is that men's income is not particularly important for family well-being. Indeed, one of the major themes in gender analyses of household dynamics is the lower proportion of income that men dedicate to their families when compared to women. Studies suggest that as a proportion of their earnings, men devote less of their income to the household and, therefore, that investing in women's income generation generally offers better returns for family well-being. For example, a study in Guatemala found that a relatively small increase in the mother's income was necessary to improve child nutrition, while an increase nearly 15 times as large was required in the father's income to produce the same benefit for children's health (Bruce et al. 1995). Similarly, in Jamaica, households without men devote a higher percentage of their income to child-specific goods (Wyss 1995).

On the surface it would appear that men are derelict in their support of children compared to women, even when employed. On the other hand, men's use of their income in social activities with male peers may be a valid effort to construct and maintain instrumental social networks, which may serve as sources of contacts and information about potential employment and provide important social support for men.

Since the early 1980s, income-generating and job creation initiatives have aimed to increase women's income in developing countries. These initiatives are, to be sure, urgently needed. But they can also reinforce the stereotype that women should and will provide for their households and that men are presumed derelict and are less involved in supporting the household. The question remains whether it is possible to promote women's income generation and at the same time to work with men to reconsider their roles and responsibilities in their households. Social policies that focus on women as the only wage-earners in a household, or as the only important wage-earners in terms of family well-being, may actually drive men away from assuming family responsibilities, serving in effect to create self-fulfilling prophecies of 'dead-beat Dads', as they have been called in the United States (Chant and Gutmann 2002; National Center on Fathers and Families (NCOFF) 2002).

Ultimately, unemployment and underemployment for men must be understood and examined beyond their economic implications. However, such considerations are rarely taken into account in social policy. For example, child support enforcement – while fundamental for women's rights and children's well-being – often takes a punitive view that men are derelict in paying child support (and in some countries makes non-payment a crime), while in many cases men are out of work for reasons beyond their control. As some advocates say, rather than 'dead-beat' Dads, many low-income fathers are 'dead-broke' Dads.

Job skills and social skills

What can young men do to improve their employment prospects? Two major factors are at play here. One is national and international market forces and economic situations that determine how many and what kind of jobs are available. Economic stagnation and trends in the workplace, notably a trend toward a reduced labour force in some sectors in some parts of the developing world, has led to too many youth chasing too few jobs. The trend toward increased employment in the informal sector has brought mixed results. Some individuals are making ends meet and even doing well in the informal market. Others, probably most, are barely making it or losing ground.

The second challenge is how an individual young man can acquire job-specific skills and social skills to improve his employability. Most experts on the issue of vocational training – and most national vocational training programmes – have concluded that young people need both technical skills or job-specific skills as well as generic social skills. The problem is that acquiring both can be a formidable challenge.

Volatile economies mean that there is often a mismatch between the skills young people have and the requirements of the workplace. In Brazil, for example, during a five-year span during the 1990s, 45 per cent of those employed in the commerce sector shifted to other economic areas, while the service sector exhibited the greatest growth. Labour markets around the world are becoming more selective, often benefiting the more experienced worker. Many of the skills needed to find and maintain work are not part of traditional vocational education programmes, many of which take a tunnel-vision approach to learning one specific, non-transferable set of skills for one kind of job. Furthermore, studies in various settings have documented that even when economies have been growing, the tendency in various employment sectors has been toward a reduced labour force, or a labour force without benefits (Teixera 1997).

Even when they exist, in most developing countries, as has been seen in previous examples, there are too few spaces in vocational training programmes. In the case of Brazil, the Ministry of Labor estimates that more than 4 million persons, adults and young people, are enrolled in some kind of vocational training nationwide. Nonetheless, they estimate that this number needs to be tripled – to reach at least 14 million persons a year – to adequately meet the demand for such training (Fundação Mauricio Sirotsky Sobrinho et al. 1997).

Apart from these trends in the workplace – the lack of jobs and the lack of places in job training programmes – there is also the lingering issue of social skills. These include traits or practices such as punctuality, communication skills, problem-solving abilities and the ability to work in a group. Previous examples have highlighted some of the difficulties that many low-income young men face in the school setting – in terms of abiding by the different norms and order that public schools generally demand. Low-income young men in many of these settings often find it difficult to show up for work on days when they do not feel like it.

In addition, many low-income young men lack role models of what a working man is like. Apart from the objective reality of too few jobs, only a minority have fathers, stepfathers or other adult men in the family who serve as role models as 'working men'. Given that most such young men have only four or five years of schooling (for young men whose average age was 16 and should have had up to ten years of education), many lack notions and habits of punctuality, perseverance and other social skills required for many formal sector jobs. They lack what Souza e Silva (2003) has called 'institutional intelligence', that is an understanding of how a given institution (the workplace) functions and a familiarity with it.

This lack of contact with working men and the lack of familiarity with the formal sector workplace probably heightens the fear that some young men express when talking about looking for work. Having little social capital for acquiring formal sector employment is both a subjective and objective barrier to finding stable employment. In other words, young men not only lack work skills but also believe that they do not fit in in a formal workplace setting. Indeed, the social codes of a formal workplace are simply unknown to many low-income young men in these settings.

Conclusions

Employment and unemployment are almost always considered to be the domains of economists. They often argue that job loss or unemployment is associated with violence, which leads to a decreased accumulation of human capital, reduced job productivity, increased absenteeism, lower earnings and lower productivity – creating a multiplier effect. While all of these associations are valid, the voices of young men suggest that there is also an identity loss or self-esteem loss multiplier effect. Loss of or lack of employment for many young men is both a lack of income and a loss of face or respect. At the same time, too many young men have never had stable employment and thus have no 'face' or respect to lose. If work is an imperative to achieve a socially recognized version of manhood, the syllogism is that no work means no manhood. It means that women will not find you attractive as long-term partners. It means that police will harass you. It means that your parents will hound you to find work. As a result, some young men turn to other ways to achieve respect or recognition – ranging from gangs, to domestic violence and substance use.

Most men, however, even those in low-income settings, are working. The question is whether the work which is available and attainable meets their needs for stable income and for status and permits them to form a family. Frequently it does not. As previously mentioned, some kinds of informal sector work, particularly itinerant sales work (selling on buses, in the street or in a marketplace), may be seen as demeaning.[3]

Young people probably require generic job-readiness skills rather than sector-specific skills. These generic skills include problem-solving abilities, basic computer literacy, communication skills, punctuality, flexibility and adaptation, among others. In many poorer countries, low-income young people do not have access to this social capital – that is, to the skills and contacts necessary to acquire employment that goes beyond subsistence. Crucial to this process is youth participation, concrete opportunities for young people to engage in the world around them in meaningful ways and in the process to acquire skills necessary for becoming skilled workers and active citizens.

Many youth development programmes worldwide – whether run by non-governmental organizations or the governmental sector – operate from a principle of busywork and are too often paternalistic. In too many cases in youth programmes, activities are defined for youth, not with them, and youth are engaged in activities that keep them busy, but often do not enhance their development. Relatively few programmes engage young people as active agents in their own development, and recognize and enhance their potential to participate fully as citizens and workers-in-training.

In addition, vocational training, income generation and micro-credit initiatives too often have unrealistic expectations of young people – that after three to six months of job training they should be able to find stable employment or create their own business. Clearly, such expectations are unrealistic for many if not most low-income youth. Many young men need immediate income and status. They need jobs, perhaps in the form of public works projects, that offer some status and immediate and stable income, while they also acquire work experience and skills for advancing in the workplace. It has become unfashionable to talk of New Deal-inspired public works and employment projects that are not 'sustainable' or that do not produce a direct and immediate financial return. But it may be precisely these kinds of job creation initiatives that are needed: employment creation that offers income in the short term, stability, status and a future and in the process allows young men to achieve the desired status of adult manhood through conventional rather than violent or illegal means.

Chapter 8

In the heat of the moment

Relating to women, having sex

Low-income heterosexual young men, like their middle-class counterparts, seek the company of young women for a variety of reasons. Some seek out young women for companionship, intimacy or sexual pleasure. Some young men establish committed relationships with women to start a family or long-term partnership. Others seek to show their male friends that they have achieved sexual conquests and mainly see women as objects for their sexual pleasure. Within these examples, there is tremendous diversity in the ways that heterosexual young men interact with and treat young women – from callous, misogynistic or *machista* at one end of the spectrum to more gender-equitable or respectful of the equal rights of young women at the other.

Frequently, however, the focus has been on the negative aspects of young men's attitudes and behaviours toward women. If the prevailing view is that low-income, urban-based young men (particularly those in *favelas* or shan-tytowns) are violent unless proven otherwise, their sexuality is often viewed in a similarly negative light. They are often seen as oversexed and promiscuous. In our laudable and necessary efforts to protect young women and girls from coerced sexual experiences, we too often group all young and adult men in a category of 'sugar daddies' (older men who pay or offer favours to younger girls for sex) or its cultural equivalent. Similarly, young men who father children at an early age are frequently stereotyped as being derelict and abdicating their paternal responsibilities, without examining the multiple reasons for their involvement, or lack thereof, in the lives of their children. Too often young men are either seen as enslaved to hormonal urges, or as sexual predators who prey on younger women and girls. In some discussions about men in Africa – the epicentre of the HIV/AIDS epidemic – the discourse is often even more inflammatory. Older men are in effect blamed for spreading HIV to younger women.

Uganda offers a telling example of negative views toward the sexuality of young men. A national law against 'defilement', referred to as having sex with a young woman under the age of 18, means that young men, themselves under age 18, are arrested and held in juvenile detention facilities if they have consensual sexual relations with a girl the same age as themselves.

To be sure, exploitative and coerced sex is too frequent and older men – who tend to have more income than younger men – are a source of HIV and other sexual health risks for many young women in Africa and elsewhere. Too many women – particularly in countries such as South Africa and Botswana – are the victims of sexual violence, which in addition to being a tremendous human rights violation, contributes to the spread of HIV. The point is that such accounts of violence against women, which must be spoken about, do not tell the entire story of heterosexual young men and their relationships with women. Too often the sexuality of young men is cast in a negative light and all young men are grouped into one large category of sexualized brutes.

Reviewing data on men's sexual behaviour worldwide, researchers at the Panos Institute in the United Kingdom estimated that 25 per cent of men worldwide carry out some sexual behaviour that puts themselves and their partners at risk for HIV/AIDS (Panos Institute 1998). While this number is significant, it means that many, perhaps most, of the world's men generally practise safer sex. While we cannot gloss over the sexual violence and unsafe sexual behaviour of a sizeable minority of the world's men, it is useful to keep this point of reference in mind.

A closer examination of the sexual and reproductive behaviour and relationship status of adolescent boys and young men suggests tremendous diversity. On average, young men around the world marry and have children later than young women. Some young men are married, but most are not; likewise, some have children, but most do not. Some are involved in mutually faithful, long-term relationships; some have sexual relations with young women and/or men outside of their primary relationships.

Young men, with the exception of parts of Africa and the Caribbean, generally have penetrative sex earlier and with more partners before forming a stable relationship than do young women. Young men are also more likely than young women to have occasional sexual partners outside of a stable relationship. The fact that many young men, married and unmarried, have multiple sexual partners has important reproductive and sexual health implications for males and females, notably regarding transmission of sexually transmitted infections (STIs), including HIV infection. This is a key rationale for seeking to understand and respond to the sexual and reproductive needs and realities of young men.

Many young men have had some sexual activity with other men, but do not define their sexual orientation by that experience. In studies around the world, between 1 per cent and 16 per cent of young men report having had some sexual contact with a male partner (Panos Institute 1998). Taboos about same-sex sexual behaviour in most of the world mean that such behaviour is often repressed, stigmatized or denied; in some countries it is also illegal. This only increases vulnerability to HIV infection and other STIs.

Some (possibly many) young men are abusive or violent toward their sexual partners, but probably most are not. Some boys and young men have themselves been victims of sexual abuse in their homes or elsewhere, most often perpetrated by other men, but also at times by women.

Some young men take a role in seeking and using condoms and other contraceptives, but many do not. Many researchers credit increased condom use among young men in some countries to HIV/AIDS prevention efforts since the late 1980s. Clearly, in some countries, increased attention to engaging young men in sexual and reproductive health seems to be having some slow impact, but more impact evaluation research is needed to confirm how widespread the changes are and the causes behind them.

How young men view women

Heterosexual young men's sexual behaviour must be seen through the lens of how they view young women. In discussions with young men in the settings discussed in this book, young men frequently showed disdain toward women and a generalized lack of respect for women. In all four areas of the world, there has been a relative relaxation of mores that discouraged young women from having sex before marriage. This trend – which translates into more young women having penetrative sex before marriage – was generally seen as negative by young men. Most young men in these settings did not believe that young women should have the same sexual freedom that they enjoyed.

Overall, male–female relationships were described as being tense and full of conflict. In Rio de Janeiro, for example, one young man said: 'these days, there's nothing [no connection and no respect] for anyone, either men or women.' Another young man in Rio de Janeiro, in a group discussion activity said: 'There are only happy endings . . . and relationships [between men and women] that last in the soap operas [on TV]. I don't know anyone here whose mother and father have been together for their whole lives.' In a group educational activity used to help encourage young men to identify characteristics of violent and non-violent intimate relationships, the group that gets selected to identify the characteristics of a relationship based on respect nearly always has trouble completing the task. A young man in one of the groups said: 'I don't know what a relationship based on respect [between a man and woman] looks like. I've never seen one.'

It is interesting to note that if many young men seem to view women as objects, rather than as individuals with rights, many young men also believe that women see them in similarly usurious ways. One young man in Chicago said:

> Personally by me being a DJ, I usually find them [women] coming after me . . . Women are pig-headed these days. If a brother has anything going for him these days [referring to work or income], girls go after him . . . They

would rather have sex with an entertainer because then they can go back to their girls and say 'I did this with blasé-blasé', you know what I'm sayin'? . . . [The kind of women I like] she's not a 'hood rat for one. That's a woman who goes with anybody . . . To me the definition of a woman is a beautiful, well-mannered, respectful, intelligent, someone with a lovely personality that does not only respect other people but has the utmost respect for herself.

(Lemar, 18, African American, in-school, non-gang-involved, Chicago)

Similarly, as we previously noted, many young men in low-income settings complained that young women in their neighbourhoods were attracted to gang-involved young men, who had access to income and status.

Another common trend among young men is that of categorizing women. Young men distinguish between girls who are seen as suitable for longer-term relationships, including marriage ('girls of faith' as young men in Rio de Janeiro called them, referring to girls they would have as their girl-friends), and 'girls of the street', referring to girls with whom they had short-term and often purely sexual relationships. In Chicago, those girls who were sexually available were called 'hood rats' and 'whores', as opposed to the 'ladies' and 'women', who were seen as marriageable. In Nigeria, those young women who had sex before marriage, either to earn income or favours or because they wanted to, were classified as 'harlots'. In much of the world, 'girls of faith' are becoming scarcer, reflecting the fact that the sexual behaviour of young women is beginning to resemble that of young men. One young man in Brazil, commenting on this trend, said: 'Young women are just giving us the other side of the same coin.'

These mostly negative attitudes toward women start even before adolescence and young adulthood. Interviews carried out with younger boys suggest that attitudes about and relationships with girls reflect both a carryover of playful competition and rivalry from childhood that characterizes boy–girl relationships in the late childhood, pre- and early adolescent phase. But they also show the beginning of the tensions found in older adolescent and adult relationships in their communities. Boys as young as 11 and 12 already show an awareness of the generally stressed nature of male–female relationships among adults and the resulting conflicts over resources and child support. Furthermore, mistrust, conflict over resources and occasional violence were reported to be common characteristics of male–female relationships, as will be discussed further in Chapter 9.

In some parts of the world, gender roles are even more polarized and girls and women are frequently described as inferior and morally weak; in some cases young women are seen as property to be given to the husband's family. Some young men criticize young women for using sex to acquire income. One group of young men (Christian and Muslim) interviewed in a secondary school in Kaduna, Nigeria, reflected these views of girls:

SALIM: A girl's burden is different. In my village [in a rural area outside Kaduna], I am from a family of four. The burden on the girl is greater. God created women to help. She is expected to do that. Here in Africa we care much more for boys than girls. Because boys remember their families, but a girl leaves the family [for her husband's family]. If there is any inconvenience for a girl, they become harlots and get what they need [they sell or trade sex for money].

EDWARD: Yes, girls may need material things more than boys and they capitalize on that [selling sex] and get what they need.

GODFRIED: Those girls are harlots. If you are a good girl, you do not lay yourself out for any man. She can learn other things, like how to sew or press hair and continue her education, and give to a man sexually at the proper time [after marriage].

NASSAR: Girls are definitely different. You [as a boy] learn how to take responsibility. That of a female, she may not have the courage to show responsibility. She may be devoted to her parents but she will leave the family and go to her husband. A boy, he will think about this future . . . but not a girl.

Nonetheless, some young men make efforts to understand the difficulties that young women face, as the following quote from a young man in Chicago suggests:

> It takes a lot to be a woman. They go through a lot of things, boy problems. I'm friends with my ex-girlfriends and they talk to me about current problems . . . Yesterday I had this girl call me . . . She just broke up with this boy . . . She wrote a letter [telling him she wanted to break up] and the guy found it and he said he was hurt so he hit her. And I told her: 'Well, didn't it hurt when he hit you?' And she was like, 'yeah'. This guy used to hit her all the time.
>
> (Dwayne, 18, African American young man, in-school, non-gang-involved, Chicago)

Some men are keenly aware of the negative treatment that women face. While their attitude may not be entirely empathetic, some men believe that the sexual harassment that women face is unjust, as did this group of adult men in Kaduna, Nigeria:

FRANKLIN: If a woman wants to get a job, she will have to give sex to get it. To become a civil servant like us, she will have to have sex.

HABIB: Unless she is not pretty or she comes from a big [powerful] family. [The rest of the men laughed at this.]

AYO: You can't let your daughter go to these places [where we work] because of these things, because you know this will happen.

FRANKLIN: Nowadays, on the police force or in the military, a woman will get promoted if she has sex. It's the natural way they work. It's in the blood of the elites to do these things.

University students in Kaduna, Nigeria, similarly reported that their university-educated female peers experienced harassment in the workplace:

SAMUEL: You [as a woman] find yourself working and you may have better experience than a man, but she has to enslave herself. Your promotion depends on getting customers and the next thing you know your boss will give you a big account. This woman I know, that happened to her. Her boss gave her a big expense account and then he asked her out on a date and he wanted to have sex with her. So she went to talk to the director of the firm and told him what had happened and he said: 'What do you think you were hired for?' Ladies are regarded as an exploitable tool.

YASSIF: At the workplace, they even tell her what to wear . . . they tell her to wear a miniskirt. She comes to your office and half her body is outside her suit. She is very beautiful and uses that . . . Her qualifications become her physique.

A few young men go beyond simply observing the unjust treatment and sexual harassment of young women and openly state that such treatment is wrong. A young Muslim man in Nigeria, for example, when his peers were criticizing women and saying that they were untrustworthy, said: 'Girls should be given the same opportunities, just as boys have.' Other young men, while usually a minority, voice a similar sense of indignation over the unfair treatment of young women.

Most young men, however, seem to be somewhere in the middle – neither completely disrespectful, nor entirely gender-equitable to the point that they criticize or question the unjust treatment of young women. To give an example, in a group of about 25 young men whom I have interacted with over several years in Brazil, there was a mixture of *machismo* and respect in their relationships with women. For example, Ronaldo, one of the young men, is described by his male and female peers as being respectful, even a gentleman in his treatment of young women, but at the same time he accepted without question the double standard that women had to remain faithful while men could have outside partners (something he said he had done).

Similarly, Murilo showed a mixture of equitable and inequitable attitudes toward young women. In one case he paid for contraception for a partner. In another instance, he helped protect a girlfriend from violence by a former boyfriend. At the same time, Murilo was sometimes verbally aggressive toward young women, calling them 'sluts' and 'whores' to their faces. João (see Chapter 3) showed tremendous dedication to his partner and child, but at the same time he believed that violence against women was justifiable in the case of her infidelity:

GB: Do you think there's any time when it's justified to hit a woman?

JOÃO: For me, you have to [hit her] if you see her going out with someone else. That deserves being hit. But if it's just an argument about day-to-day things, you didn't do this, so I'll hit you, I told you to do it and you didn't, for me that's no justification. Only if she goes out with someone else and you find her with the other guy. If it's not that, it's just cowardice to hit her.

In summary, some young men are struggling to be respectful in their relationships with women. Some seem to be rehearsing or beginning to have longer-term relationships with women based on a reasonable degree of mutual respect. It is difficult to predict whether these young men will be respectful and more gender-equitable in the long run in their adult, intimate relationships. For some, it seems likely that they will be respectful, particularly if their female partners also have the means to demand respect – which often implies that she has her own income or contributes to household income. For others, there are signs that they are already repeating some of the sexist attitudes they observed in their own homes.

Male–female relationships in many low-income, urban settings are fraught with mistrust and conflict (and too often with violence). While part of this tension may be related to the stress associated with poverty, much of it is also rooted in the double standard around sexual fidelity. Too many men (lower and middle income) accept and defend the double standard that they are allowed outside sexual partners, while their girlfriends and wives are not. Many young men say they monitor the whereabouts of their girlfriends, and complain if their girlfriends are out with 'loose' friends. At the same time, young women are frequently convinced that their boyfriends and husbands have an outside partner – and many do, but some do not. And as previously mentioned, many young men say they have rarely if ever seen a male–female relationship based on respect. These tendencies make it difficult to be optimistic, in the short run anyway, about the state of male–female relationships in many parts of the world.

But there are also examples of positive and trusting interchanges, even if few in number. For example, Jamaican researchers Janet Brown and Barry Chevannes (1998) conclude based on research throughout the English-speaking Caribbean that while male–female relationships among low-income couples are often characterized by mistrust, others include sharing, equity, mutual respect and healthy doses of humour. Thus, although poverty and rigid gender roles often create conflict, tension and mistrust between couples – and though gender inequities often overshadow examples of mutual respect – there are examples of cooperation in male–female relationships which often escape our research.

The meaning of sex to boys and young men

Where does sex fit into this equation? What does sex mean to young men? As previously mentioned, in most of the world, young men generally have penetrative sex earlier and with more partners before forming a relationship than do young women, although since the 1980s there has been a general approximation between the median age of first vaginal intercourse between boys and girls (Singh et al. 2000). After forming relationships, young men are also more likely than young women to have occasional sexual partners outside these relationships.

Apart from the timing, the meaning of early sexual activity is often different for boys than for girls. Young men often view sexual initiation as a way to prove that they are 'men', that is to affirm their identity, and to have status in the male peer group (Marsiglio 1988). In interviews with lower-income and lower-middle-income young men in Rio de Janeiro, having had sex (heterosexual sex) and acquiring employment were seen as the two milestones for becoming a man (Barker and Loewenstein 1997). For many young men, penetrative sex – which is often considered the only 'sex that counts' – is seen as an accomplishment and something to acquire and show off, like a merit badge or certificate of manhood.

In some parts of the world, some young men have their first sexual encounter and subsequent sexual encounters with a sex worker, in part at least to affirm their manhood before the male peer group. In Thailand, 61 per cent of young men report having had sex with a sex worker at least once (Im-em 1998). In Argentina, 42 per cent of secondary school boys interviewed in one study said their first sexual experience was with a sex worker (Necchi and Schufer 1998). In India, between 19 per cent and 78 per cent of men report having had sex with a sex worker (Jejeebhoy 1996).

Young men may be encouraged to have sex with sex workers by male family members or peers. Indeed in most such sexual encounters and sexual initiation with sex workers, young men go in groups, and frequently out of a sense of obligation to fulfil a socially proscribed role. Clearly, many young men experience sexual pleasure in their early sexual experiences, with sex workers or other partners, but it is important to affirm the pressure that young men experience to demonstrate sexual prowess. This pressure and these rigid social 'scripts' show similarities even in the most diverse of settings.

Pakistan is an overwhelmingly Muslim country where traditional mores of sexual behaviour are widespread; young women are expected to remain chaste until marriage, and in rural areas, women have been killed by family members for sexual transgressions. In the heart of the old walled city of Lahore is a red-light district that has reportedly functioned in the same place for more than five centuries. It is dutifully opened and closed every night by police. Most of the men who go there are younger. Frequently, they walk in pairs, holding hands (a common demonstration of friendship among men). A common joke circulating goes like this:

> A young man has just got married and he is finally alone with his bride. When the time comes for them to have sex, he makes a call on a cordless phone. He calls up his male friends and says: 'What do I do now?'

The clear intention in the joke is to show the shameful inexperience of the young man on his wedding night. A 'real man', they implied, would know what to do. These subtle and not-so-subtle pressures are behind many young men's first sexual experiences – in Pakistan and elsewhere. Some boys may not be ready or may not want this kind of sexual initiation. In addition, early sexual experiences with sex workers may contribute to lasting patterns in which men believe that women should serve them sexually. Few young men report these first sexual experiences with sex workers as being tremendous sexual encounters. Most young men describe feeling scared, and afterwards, relieved.

These are important points to highlight in thinking about young men's sexuality. Indeed various studies find that boys often share their heterosexual conquests with pride with the male peer group, while doubts or lack of sexual experience and any homosexual experiences are hidden or denied. Not having become sexually active, and sometimes having just one female partner, can be motives for ridicule in the male peer group.

Many young men lie about or exaggerate their sexual experience before their male peers, particularly if they have never had penetrative sex with a woman. Some young men are able to articulate the stress they suffer by direct pressure from their male peer group to have sexual relations. In a study in Guinea, West Africa, boys said they worried that if they did not have sex with a girl, their reputation would suffer among their male peers (Gorgen et al. 1998). In a similar vein, one young man in Chicago said this:

> I mean, I never had sex with a girl. My friends, you know, ask me about it and I lie about it. I know it ain't right [to lie to them] . . . [sometimes] I just tell them I'm proud to be a virgin 'cause I'm not walkin' around with no disease. They tell me I'm a punk . . . but I'm like I'm not worried about that. It may come across my mind sometimes. Like if I get this picture in my head of my friends . . . they just sittin' there laughin' and makin' fun of me and I think, man, I wish that hadn't been me [telling them I never had sex].
>
> (Marvin, 15, African American, in-school, non-gang-involved, Chicago)

Another young man in Rio de Janeiro showed considerable shame about not having had penetrative sex by the age of 16. In one discussion, he said he had sex once when he was 10 or 11. Later, he admitted that he had not had sex, but felt ashamed to admit it. He said that when his male peers get together, they frequently discuss sex: 'They say it was great [having sex] with so-and-so and who they want to have sex with but, I don't know, I don't say anything, I just let them talk.'

A group of younger African American boys (aged 11–14) in Chicago reflected this pressure as well:

RUPERT: Some [boys start their sexual activity] at like age 13. They try to get a head start on us.

JAMES: We're too young [to start having sex]. We should wait until we're 16.

RUPERT: They [his peer group] would call me a faggot if I say that. They tell me: 'You need to get some' [have sex with a girl].

In summary, while it is true that the first sexual encounters of young men are more likely than those of young women to be self-willed, there is frequently social pressure involved. The pressure on boys is, of course, far different than overt coercion and sexual abuse and violence that young women more frequently report in many parts of the world. Nonetheless, the social pressure that many boys report calls attention to the question of whether boys have their first sexual encounters for their own pleasure and curiosity – or to fulfil a proscribed social role.

Young men and sex in Rio de Janeiro's *favelas*

In Rio de Janeiro, *baile funk* (funk dances) are popular in *favelas*. They are arguably the focal point of social life – and sexual life – for young people in *favelas*, blasting a sexually charged mixture of funk, hip hop, techno and rap on weekend nights in many low-income neighbourhoods around the city. Young men often meet girlfriends and occasional sexual partners at the dances.

The music is deafening; conversation is all but impossible. Many youth are dancing; nearly all the dance steps consist of pelvic thrusts and simulations of sexual intercourse. During one song, a young woman of 15 sings about how much girls from the *favela* adore sex. The lyrics say that all the girls from the *favela* like 'it' in the mouth, the vagina, the anus, and like it all the time.

Young men, usually in groups of two or three, roam the main dance floor area. By about 3:00 a.m. there may be 300 to 400 young people inside. The dances typically last until the break of day. In the later hours, some young men say, sex takes place in the dark corners of the open space.

A few weeks later in another *favela*, a group of young men and young women were arguing about funk dances in their community. The young men were defensive about the dances. They say that some dances have fighting, while others do not. One young man said that while group sex takes place at some of the dances, others are 'calm'. Several young women immediately questioned this, saying that when they go to the dances, guys pass their hands on their bodies without asking or insinuate openly that they want to have sex. Some of the young men countered by saying that girls go voluntarily to the dances and often dress provocatively when they do. One young woman defended her right to dress however she wants without that implying that any boy who wants can touch her.

The funk dances have been criticized by the media, the police, community leaders and now in this case, by young women. A recent series of newspaper articles had alleged that girls were becoming pregnant during unprotected group sex at some funk dances, or had contracted sexually transmitted diseases during sex with multiple partners at the dances. Responding to this, one young man we spoke with said: 'Everyone wants to blame the funk dances for this . . . as if girls didn't get pregnant before.'

A study in one *favela* found that nearly half of young people (boys and girls) aged 13–19 surveyed said they frequent the funk dances, and among those, 65 per cent go at least three times a month. In another study, more than half of young men interviewed said they were at the funk dance or another similar space in the community immediately before their last sexual encounter. Whatever one says about the funk dances, they are the place to be for most young people on the weekend and they are the centre of young people's sexual activity. Young people go to the dances to see and be seen. Sexual partnering is public knowledge. Frequently after the dances, young men can be heard talking about who 'went' (had sex) with whom. Those young men who did not follow through with an initial conversation with a young woman would be chided for 'going soft in the heat of the moment'.

It is difficult to imagine more diverse settings than the old walled city of Lahore and Rio de Janeiro's *favelas*, but similarities hold. In both settings, young men seek sexual conquests before the watchful and judging eyes of their male peers. Their sexual encounters take place in close range of male friends who will confirm and affirm the 'score'. 'Chickening out' or not knowing what to do or say in the heat of the moment may result in ridicule.

Indeed, while the funk dances in Rio's *favelas* represent a culturally specific setting, similar dynamics play out in bars and dance halls in the Caribbean, elsewhere in Latin America, and many urban centres in Africa. Young men in these settings often say they do not take their girlfriends to such places; typically they are looking for occasional sexual partners. (However, in some cases, a girl they meet in such settings can become a stable partner.) Many of the young men also have stable partners or steady girlfriends. Said one young man in Rio de Janeiro: 'The rice and beans [the daily staple] is at home [with my steady girlfriend] . . . At the dance, it's the filet mignon.'

In such settings, many young men say they know they should use condoms, but often do not or do not use them consistently. Sexual encounters, the young men say, are spontaneous and opportunistic. 'You never know when you will get lucky,' one said. In the 'heat of the moment', several young men said, 'you know you should use a condom, but you don't have one, or can't be bothered.' Alcohol, marijuana and other substances are frequently part of the equation – a way to loosen up and overcome shyness.

At the dances and bars, gender plays out in mostly traditional ways: young men pursue women. In some dance halls and bars in the four countries included here, some young women have sex in exchange for money, drinks or gifts. But it would be an oversimplification to say that only young men want or pursue sex. Some young women also affirm their sexual desires and sexual initiative. One young woman in Brazil said: 'If my boyfriend can go to the funk dances, so can I.'

Sex in the era of AIDS

The funk dance highlights some of the challenges of encouraging safer sex among low-income young men. Rates of HIV in the four regions studied range from less than 1 per cent of the adult population in the case of Brazil, the United States and the English-speaking Caribbean to nearly 10 per cent in the case of Nigeria. Rates of other sexually transmitted infections are even higher. Among the youth population (ages 15–24) in the four countries, HIV rates are 0.64 per cent for men and 0.48 per cent for women in Brazil, 0.82 per cent for young men and 0.85 per cent for young women in Jamaica, 3 per cent for young men and 5.85 per cent for women in Nigeria and 0.48 per cent for young men and 0.23 per cent for young women in the United States (UNFPA 2003). In the case of sub-Saharan Africa as a whole, young women represent 67 per cent of HIV/AIDS cases among the 15–24 population, compared to 31 per cent in Latin America and the Caribbean and 33 per cent in industrialized countries. In the case of South Asia, young women represent 62 per cent of persons living with HIV/AIDS in the 15–24 age group (UNFPA 2003).

Nonetheless, if changing young men's sexual behaviour is complex, there are some positive signs. For example, condom use among young men in Brazil, and much of Latin America, has increased since the early 1990s but is still inconsistent, and varies according to the reported nature of the partner or relationship (e.g., occasional, regular, sex worker). National data on condom use in Brazil found that in 1986 fewer than 5 per cent of young men reported using a condom during first sexual intercourse, compared to nearly 50 per cent in 1999 (UNAIDS 1999). In the United States, reported condom use among young men aged 13–19 more than doubled from about one-fifth in 1979 to more than half (57.5 per cent) in 1998. But only 35 per cent said they had used a condom every time they had sex (Sonenstein et al. 1995).

At least part of this increase in condom use is related to changing peer group norms and community norms related to increased awareness about HIV/AIDS. Nonetheless, there are still several challenges and barriers to promoting young men's increased condom use. These include the sporadic nature of their sexual activity, lack of information on correct use, reported discomfort, social norms that inhibit communication between partners and rigid norms about whose responsibility it is to propose condom use. In many settings because sexual and reproductive health is seen to be a 'female' concern, women must suggest condom use or other contraceptive methods. At the same time, prevailing norms frequently hold that it is the man's responsibility to acquire condoms, since for a young woman to carry condoms would suggest that she 'planned' to have sex.

One of the results of inconsistent condom use by young men is high rates of sexually transmitted infections. A study we carried out with 749 men aged 15–60 in three neighbourhoods in Rio de Janeiro (two low income, one middle income) found that 15 per cent of all men reported having had an STI at least once, but only 42 per cent said they informed their partner about it (Instituto Promundo and Instituto Noos 2003). Other studies have confirmed that young men have high rates of STIs, and sometimes do not seek treatment or rely on self-treatment.[1]

Studies in other settings have found similarly high rates of STIs. For some STIs, men show no symptoms, meaning they can pass the infection to their partner without knowing. Research carried out by the World Health Organization (1995), for example, in a variety of countries finds that an increasing number of young males are contracting chlamydial urethritis, which is asymptomatic in men in up to 80 per cent of cases. Research in South Korea found that 17 per cent of male industrial workers (average age 25.3) and 3 per cent of students (average age 22.1) reported that they had had in the past or presently had an STI (Senderowitz 1995). Studies in the United States have found that 10–29 per cent of sexually active teenage girls and 10 per cent of teenage boys who were tested for STIs had chlamydia (Alan Guttmacher Institute 1998).

Many existing HIV prevention campaigns have focused on raising awareness or imparting information about HIV. Yet research has consistently confirmed that having accurate information about HIV is insufficient to lead to behaviour change. This gap between knowledge and behaviour suggests a continuing resistance to condom use and other safer sex practices based in large part on how boys and young men view gender roles and sexual activity.

In some settings, for example, young men believe that risky or unprotected sex is the only sex 'that counts'. In a study in 14 countries, the most common reason males reported for not using condoms was that condoms reduce sexual pleasure (Finger 1998). Some men and women believe that men's need for sex is uncontrollable, and that sex is better when it is unplanned. Some men say that they cannot turn down any opportunity to have sex, even if they do not have a condom, because it would compromise their sense of manhood (Aramburu and Rodriguez 1995; Barker and Loewenstein 1997).

All of this implies that successfully promoting safer sex behaviour, particularly condom use, requires engaging boys and young men in thoughtful discussions about gender stereotypes and sexual behaviour and attitudes – more than just mere information provision.

What boys want to know

There is a tremendous amount of research on youth and sexual information, attitudes and behaviour related to reproductive and sexual health and HIV/AIDS. Most of this research has focused on the problem behaviours of young men, or cast them in a negative light. There has been relatively little discussion of how boys feel about sexuality and the many doubts they have, including those related to pubertal changes.

Boys generally go through puberty between the ages of 10 and 13, when hormonal changes drive physical changes, including the production of sperm. Most boys have nocturnal emissions or 'wet dreams' during this period. Many boys have doubts or questions about these body changes, but are generally not encouraged to talk about them. In some cases boys may be given more information about women's bodies than about their own. When we discourage boys from talking about their bodies and sexual health at early ages, we may be starting lifelong difficulties for men in talking about sex – outside the context of sexual conquests.

Masturbation is frequently part of the early – and ongoing – sexual lives of young men, although it too is rarely talked about and, if so, generally to be ridiculed. Only in a few enlightened sexuality education programmes has masturbation been openly discussed, and presented in a positive light, for example, by representing a way for young men to come to understand their bodies and their sexual pleasure, or as an alternative to penetrative sex.

Most young men in the settings described in this book have had some kind of sexuality education, generally in school, but nearly universally this information was described as much less useful than what they learned about sex on the street, with friends, extended family members or with sexual partners. Indeed, many young men said they learned more 'on their own' about sex than they did in the classroom setting. Furthermore, in terms of the age that sex education is taught, many young men say that it is taught far too late:

> It [the sex education course I had] was too late ... it was eighth grade. I mean, come on. I was in fourth, fifth, sixth grade when I had sex, way before eighth ... You can't compare generations of the past [to us] 'cause for the generation of the past, sex was something sacred. Now sex is like a basket-ball game, everybody want to play the game but not everybody know how to play the game ... You learn about sex on your own, like drivin' a car.
>
> (Julius, 18, African American, in-school, non-gang-involved, Chicago)

Significantly, most sexuality education programmes focus on reproduction and contraception, yet adolescent boys and young men frequently say they want to know about or discuss masturbation, penis size, sexual relations and its various forms, sexual 'performance', and female sexuality. Indeed, when boys and young men are asked what they would like to know about sexuality, they frequently want to discuss sexual pleasure, how to satisfy a partner and how girls and women 'think'. One young man who partici-pated in a group educational project for young men carried out by Instituto Promundo in Brazil said that his male peers ridiculed him for participating in the group, saying it was for 'wimps'. But when he told them that the ses-sions gave him information about sex and about how to sexually please a female partner, several of his peers wanted to join the group. Indeed, infor-mation about female anatomy and the female sexual response is generally also seen as an important area of competence, as this 13-year-old African American in Chicago suggests here:

JAMES: In [this sexuality education group] ... we talk about puberty and where a girl's hole is at, where a boy's hole is.
GB: Is that useful to know?
JAMES: Yeah, it's good so you'll know ... like that girls have three holes so you won't make a fool of yourself [when you have sex with a girl].

Conclusions

Sexuality education and HIV/AIDS prevention efforts, of course, must include accurate information, but they must also take place in settings where young men and boys can present their concerns and doubts without being criticized or ridiculed. They should include discussions about young women and their needs, realities and ways of viewing the world. Indeed, the most successful sexuality education and HIV/AIDS prevention programmes for young men promote a critical reflection with them – enhancing their ability to question sexist norms, and the social pressure they face to live up to these.

Discussions with young men who show more gender-equitable atti-tudes and behaviour suggest that they have become highly critical and reflective about gender norms and thus feel confident to question or ignore the pressure or chiding they experience from peers. They have assumed their sexuality as their own, as opposed to being on display for judgment by their male peers. They have learned – sometimes the hard way – to empathize with women, and are thus more attuned to their partner's needs and well-being. Murilo, who was introduced in Chapter 5, showed this kind of reflection:

> A lot of guys will have a girlfriend, then they'll go and cheat on her. So then later when they want to find a girlfriend, it'll be difficult. Because then the girls will think: 'Does this guy want to be with me and then he'll go with someone else?' So then girls don't want to go out with him. So then the guy will start to think and he'll go slowly. He'll start going out with just one girl.
>
> (Murilo, 17, African Brazilian, Rio de Janeiro)

In the face of the trends described here, from Pakistan to Rio de Janeiro's *favelas*, promoting this kind of critical reflection may seem utopic. Nonetheless, diverse groups from Africa to Latin America have been able to engage with young men in processes like this. In Nigeria, for example, young men who participated with an organization called Conscientizing Male Adolescents, reported this:

> I used to believe that when a girl says no it is yes. This was the belief in my mind and those of my friends. [We believed that] when we play together and touch a woman's sensitive parts, she says no but she enjoys it. Through the program . . . I learned how to listen to girls . . . [since then] I have talked to friends, cousins [about this topic].

Similarly, in Brazil, work has led to the development of an initiative called Program H – Engaging Young Men in the Promotion of Health and Gender Equity – which works both in group educational settings and at the community levels, to change individual attitudes and community norms about what it means to be a man. Evaluation of the Program H activities has demonstrated measurable changes in attitudes on the part of young men who participate, including more flexible views about gender, increased reported condom use and a decline in self-reported symptoms of sexually transmitted infections among participants (see the Appendix for more information). One young man who participated said:

> I learned to talk more with girlfriend. Now I worry more about her [worry about what she likes sexually and how she feels]. Our sex life is better . . . it's important to know what the other persons wants, listen to them. Before [the workshops], I just worried about myself.
>
> (Marcelo, 19, African Brazilian, Rio de Janeiro)

This young man's girlfriend confirmed that he had in fact started to talk to her more, to listen to when and how she wanted to have sexual relations, and to see that having sex was not the only important part of their relationship.

In our laudable desire for immediate solutions, the recent focus in the field of HIV/AIDS and sexual and reproductive health has been high-technology based: microbicides, anti-retroviral medicines and vaccines.[2] Some solutions will be found through these high-tech and medically driven initiatives. But no medication nor prophylactic device will reduce men's violence against women, nor will microbicides guarantee that young men treat women well and become empathetic partners who care for their own health and the health of their partners. Changing young men's attitudes and behaviours so as to promote true and lasting gender equality is often a slow process. It includes fomenting changes at the broader social level as well as working with young people directly. Ultimately this is as dramatic and effective as a vaccine when a young man participating in such processes goes from seeing women as sexual objects to seeing them as equals.

Chapter 9

Learning to live with women, becoming fathers

Beyond their first sexual relationships, how do young men live, coexist and form long-term relationships and families with women? What are these relationships like? Is violence involved? And what about those young men who are fathers? It is useful to start this reflection with a discussion of the general nature of young men's more stable relationships with women. As seen in Chapter 8, most young men have a longer period of sexual experimentation than young women, more partners before forming a stable relationship, and more occasional partners (and even regular, outside partners) even when in stable relationships.

From hanging out to stable relationships

When do young men begin to move from more casual sexual relationships to longer-term, committed relationships? What factors are involved? These are often the burning questions that young women ask about young men. Indeed, situation comedies, talk shows and women's magazines around the world frequently tell stories of heterosexual young men who seek purely casual relationships and shun responsibility and commitment. In coffee shops and bars around the world, the complaints of middle-class, heterosexual young women are often related to men's supposed unwillingness to commit themselves. In poorer parts of the world, there is a similar discourse: men are untrustworthy, seek quantity over quality in their intimate relationships or make a woman pregnant and then leave.

These tendencies do of course exist; some, perhaps many, young men show these characteristics. And, as we saw in Chapter 8, the social pressure on young men to prove their sexual prowess is clearly related to the difficulties with intimacy and commitment that some men experience.

In their early twenties, most young men in the settings described in this book begin to form more stable relationships. In Chicago, Rio de Janeiro and parts of the Caribbean, more often than not, the relationships they establish are common law, at least initially. In the case of Nigeria, most of these more stable relationships are within the context of marriage. In all of these settings, the timing of this first, more stable relationship often involves either one or two factors: an unplanned pregnancy and having income or a job.

Reports and seminars organized by the World Health Organization and other organizations in 2002 have focused on arranged and sometimes forced marriages on younger women. But to what extent is marriage for young men purely a matter of free choice? While research on young men's experiences of partner selection is limited, particularly within settings where arranged marriages are common, it is worth questioning the assumption that young men have freedom in their selection of spouses or the timing of their first stable relationships.

Researchers working in India suggest that while boys and men are undoubtedly privileged compared to their sisters, their two most significant life decisions – choice of occupation and that of their mate – are, like women, largely decided by adults in the family rather than being purely a matter of personal choice (Shweder 2003). Discussions with young men in a variety of settings suggest that young men (and adult men), experience significant pressure from family in terms of their choice of mate and the timing of their marriages.

This pressure, of course, has different ramifications and men nearly everywhere have a greater ability to operate in the public realms of schooling and the workplace, which provides them with some 'room to manoeuvre' when subjected to family pressure. Nonetheless, it is pertinent to ask how much choice young men experience in choosing partners and having children in some parts of the world.

Men in Nigeria, for example, report pressure from their families to marry or to have children; at the same time, they said they are delaying marriage so they can complete their education and improve their work prospects, as with these university students in Kaduna, Nigeria:

JOHN: Some families want to know if you are a man. They want to know if you are man enough to handle a woman, in bed I mean. And so they will say: 'You have all these beautiful women around you, why don't you think about getting married. Can't you handle them?'

AYO: Yeah, if you are not talking about women [with your family], they may think you are impotent or something . . . you have to have a strategy [to convince your family that you are interested in women].

Others say:

ALFRED: In some parts of the southwest of Nigeria [where he was from], you [as a man] have to prove your fertility before you get married. You have to get a girl pregnant before you are married to prove that you are a man.

YUSSIF: You know the truth is, we get married to have children . . . you prove yourself to your family by how many children you have. You know, your mother will say that she wants to have grandchildren.

Here, marriage and childbearing are as much about satisfying others – particularly their families – as about young men's own desires for family formation. As in the case of their sexual activity – which is often 'performed' for the approval of others – for young men, family formation and having children is often related to satisfying the expectations of others.

Educational attainment is heralded as one of the major factors, if not *the* major factor, influencing age at marriage and childbearing, both for boys and girls. What is the relationship between schooling and age at marriage for young men? Enrolment in school, meaningful work, and access to savings or some form of financial independence have been linked to, and promoted as, ways for delaying marriage in parts of the world where girls often marry young. Indeed, there is considerable evidence that higher levels of educational attainment are associated with lower rates of early childbearing and early marriage among young men as well as women.

However, for most young men, work is the chief basis of their identity, or the main cultural requisite for achieving manhood. For a young man, being able to support oneself and one's family financially is generally a precursor to form a family. Thus, achieving the provider role – acquiring gainful employment – is a signal event for many young males to begin childbearing. Accordingly, many young men in low-income settings seek to start families or more stable relationships but feel that they cannot because of their lack of income and work. They are in effect trapped in a perpetual boyhood, seeking to be men – and to form families – but unable to acquire employment and status. In these circumstances, they may either avoid more stable relationships or are not attractive to women as potential mates.

Stress, violence and the nature of male–female relationships

Chapter 8 described the general sense of mistrust in many male–female relationships. It is worth repeating that most young men say they do not know what a healthy, democratic relationship between a man and a woman looks like. Put it another way: many young men lack internal working models of what healthy, caring and respectful intimate relationships look like. Most young people are not adequately prepared for learning how to peacefully coexist and cohabit in stable, satisfying intimate relationships. This begs the question of how much societies prepare young men or young women for some of their most important relationships. Indeed, if we see young men's relationships with young women as setting the tone for the kinds of relationships these young men will have later in life, then the basic atmosphere of distrust is troubling – because of what it means for present relationships and for future families, the care of children, and the quality of life of young men and women.

Young men and women often say that in dating, 'things' are less serious, and conflicts less frequently lead a young man to use physical violence. However, once a couple is cohabiting and has children, which often happens between the ages of 20 and 24, the first experiences of living together are often reported to be stressful and fraught with conflict. Many young men, as a result, report that they use physical violence against their partners. This violence emerged, they say, when the woman did not 'fulfil her part of the bargain'. This might include not taking care of children, not taking care of the house, spending too much time with her friends, or when there is suspicion of sexual infidelity.

Older men in some settings suggest that over time, they learn how to cohabit with women in less physically violent ways. It is clear from numerous studies that older women report higher lifetime rates of victimization by physical violence. However, it may be that early in relationships, young men's use of violence against women is more commonplace than among older men. There may be a developmental trajectory of individuals and relationships, and that time spent together, along with maturation of the individual, may contribute to less physically violent cohabitation for some couples.[1]

Unfortunately, physical violence is all too commonplace in many relationships. Most research on violence against women has focused on adult couples and women, but some studies suggest that patterns of violence in heterosexual relationships emerge in early relationships. For example, studies of high school and college students in New Zealand and the United States found that between 20 per cent of young men and 59 per cent of young women have experienced physical aggression during a dating relationship (Jezl et al. 1996; Magdol et al. 1997).

There is a growing body of studies showing the extent of men's violence against women. In a mid-1990s review, more than 30 studies from around the world show that between one-fifth and one-half of women interviewed have been subject to physical violence by a male partner (Heise 1994). In a 1993 national survey in Barbados, 30 per cent of women aged 20–45 reported having been beaten as adults and 50 per cent of men and women interviewed say their mother was beaten. In Colombia, a national sample found that one in five women said they had been physically abused and one in ten reported having been raped by their husbands (Heise 1994). A national study in Nicaragua found that 29 per cent of women said they had been physically or sexually abused by a male partner; in 57 per cent of the cases children were present at the time of violence and in 36 per cent of cases, the violence happened when the woman was pregnant (Alatorre 2002).

Men's violence against women is so commonplace in some settings that it becomes banal, unworthy of special attention; in some places, violence in intimate relationships is described as ubiquitous. Said one young man in Brazil: 'My mother takes some hits everyday from her boyfriend . . . Sometimes they fight, then they get back together. That's how it is.' Said another young man:

> Whatever we may feel about it [a man hitting a woman], we can only watch . . . [we] can't do anything. It's their problem. Shit, do what? She got beat up . . . I've seen lots of these fights before. I've seen guys try to get involved and getting punched in the face. Like we'll defend the woman . . . then afterwards, the woman will be all hugging him again.
>
> (Reginaldo, 18, African Brazilian, Rio de Janeiro)

The causes and factors associated with men's use of violence against women are multiple, complex and interwoven. Clearly, the reasons or underlying factors are rooted in the way that manhood is constructed, that is, what it means to be a man. For some men, violence represents an attempt to maintain traditional gender roles, of trying to keep a woman trapped in her traditional role (de Keizjer 1995). In other cases, physical violence is seen as a valid way for men to express emotions or frustrations – since men are not 'allowed' to show emotions in other ways (Kaufman 1993; Nolasco 1993).

Work in the Caribbean and from Brazil has found that domestic violence is often seen as part of the informal rules of cohabitation. If the man sustains the household, the woman is expected to take care of the house and be sexually faithful to him. Violation of this 'contract' on the part of the woman is seen by many men and women as grounds or justification for physical violence. When the roles are reversed and women sustain the household, some women may become physically violent toward men (Brown et al. 1995; Barker and Loewenstein 1997).

Studies in the United States have found that domestic violence is linked to economic stress, low self-esteem (on the part of the victim and the perpetrator) and traditional ideas about gender roles (Tauchen et al. 1991). Research we coordinated in Brazil found that men's use of physical violence against women is related to low levels of educational attainment, traditional views about masculinity and having witnessed or experienced physical violence in their own home as a child (Instituto Promundo and Instituto Noos 2003).

Many young men justify their use of violence against women by saying that women provoke violence, either by not respecting a man's temper or by slapping him, which was described as the most common form of women's violence toward men. For some young men we have spoken with, it seemed to be a logical consequence of women being manipulative that men resort to violence against them. In some settings, the general tone of male–female relationships was described as violent, with both men and women using violence against each other, as 17-year-old Darryl, an African American in Chicago, explained:

DARRYL: I think that's stupid [to hit girls]. Why hit on a female? If you bigger than her, or even if you not bigger, that's disrespectful. If you get mad, even if she hits you, you have to just walk away.

GB: Do a lot of guys hit girls?

DARRYL: Yeah, a lot of guys, they hit back [if a girl hits them] regardless of who it is. So far what I observed is that if girls hit boys, security [guards at school] breaks it up before the guy can hit back. I hear girls say that if he hit 'em, they [the girl] gonna kill him . . . they say they cut 'em and all that but I ain't seen it happen.

Said one 19-year-old man in Rio de Janeiro:

> I mean, look [when a man hits a woman], the woman did something to get the guy [angry] . . . She did something, let's suppose, that gave him a reason to hit her . . . She slipped up . . . treated the guy badly. Maybe he let it go for a while. Then there was some moment when he couldn't take it anymore, so he beat the shit out of her . . . so you're going to let it go when you see that she treated him badly.

In addition to individual and relationship factors, how cultures generally view violence against women is also linked to whether men use such violence. Some societies or cultures are more accepting, even encouraging, of men's use of violence against women. A cross-cultural study or comparison between 90 societies found that those cultures which had the high rates of gender-based violence generally had authoritarian styles in the household, male dominance in general and a widespread acceptance of physical violence (Levinson 1989). Indeed, even in settings where only a minority of men carry out physical violence against women, there is considerable support for men's use of violence against women. To give an example, in survey research in low-income areas in Brazil, about one in four men surveyed reported having used physical violence against a woman in his most recent stable relationships but up to two-thirds of young men believed that violence was acceptable against women when a woman 'cheats on him' (Instituto Promundo and Instituto Noos 2003).

Men's use of violence against women is learned, and passed from one generation to the next. Various studies have found that having witnessed or been a victim of violence in the home is associated with using violence against a close partner. Indeed, it is clear that children are frequently present when men use violence against women and are victims of men's violence. In one study, children were present in more than half of the most recent incidents of men's use of violence against women (Instituto Promundo and Instituto Noos 2003). In the same study, 40 per cent of men said they had witnessed violence by a man against a woman in their home of origin and 45.5 per cent reported having been victims of physical violence in their homes.

Men's use of violence against women has direct implications for the next generation of boys and girls. Boys grow up believing that such violence is normal and justified, while girls may grow up thinking that they must accept it, as the following quote illustrates:

> With my wife, one time I got to the point that I hit her. It was something that came from my youth. I was desperate . . . I felt everything I went through when I was young. I saw my father [hit my mother and us]. If you didn't listen to him or do what he wanted, he started hitting. One day, when I had said everything I could and I didn't have anything else to say, I hit her.
>
> (Luis, 19, Hispanic, Chicago).

What about the young men who do not use violence against women in settings where support for violence is high? Where do they come from? If it is the case that up to a third or more of men have used physical violence against women, there are many men who abhor such violence, even in settings where it is prevalent. Some young men say they would never be violent toward women because they had learned in their own households that this was not proper behaviour. Said one young man in Chicago: 'I can't hit a girl. It don't feel right. If you hit a girl you like don't have no courage.' Another young man said:

> You know, sometimes I get real mad at a girl to the limit and I just feel like crushing her . . . but I know how I was raised. I was raised not to hit girls. My mother, she had these fights with this one guy but she never got beat up. You know, it ain't like that [in my family] so why would I go out and do this to a person?
>
> (Michael, 18, African American, Chicago)

For some young men, having been violent or abusive toward a girl or a woman and then having repented or 'seen the errors of their ways' is an important personal experience that can contribute to being non-violent toward women:

> I used to be in that stuff [gangs] but not anymore. And girls used to come up to me by the dozens 'cause I had money and cars . . . I made a reputation for myself that will pass for myself over a long time. Even when I'm older people will still look at me and say 'aren't you that rapper . . . You were the boy who were representing as a dog, you did bad things to girls.' I was going

> out with this one girl and she made me mad and I left her in the street . . . If I ever have a son, I'm gonna teach him that that's not how you treat women.
>
> (Wayne, 18, African American, Chicago)

Said another young man when asked who taught him not to hit girls:

> My father, my auntie, my great auntie, all the people I live with [told me not to hit girls]. And then one time I hit a girl when I was in the fifth grade . . . We was playing baseball and I tagged her . . . and she slapped me and I slapped her back. And even today she got a mark on her face from where I slapped her and I felt bad about that so I just made myself a promise that I would never do that again.
>
> (Chuckie, 18, African American, Chicago)

Other factors associated with young men's questioning of violence against women include having seen the negative effects of this violence first hand, for example having seen a father or stepfather use violence against a mother. One young man in Brazil had seen his mother experience partial hearing loss as a result of his stepfather's violence. This event led him to write a play about violence to engage other men on the issue. For other young men, it was key that a woman in the family – a mother or grandmother – expelled a violent man from the household. In some cases, such actions sent clear messages to young men that such violence was not to be tolerated. And, for young men who have seen fathers and stepfathers treat women with respect rather than violence, such violence generally is seen as abhorrent.

These examples offer insights for formulating strategies to reduce men's violence against women. Since the early 1980s in many developing countries, laws against men's violence against women have been enacted, and considerable effort has gone into keeping women safe once they have experienced such violence. In a few countries, programmes are also beginning to work with young men to prevent gender-based violence. In Brazil, a coalition of organizations engage groups of young men in low-income communities to work as peer health promoters, who reach out to other young men with messages about gender violence prevention and gender equality. An outreach campaign, called In the Heat of the Moment Campaign, which is part of the project has engaged well-known male rap singers to question violence against women. In Canada, the White Ribbon Campaign was founded as a movement of men questioning other men about violence against women and has since spread to more than 30 countries. In the United States, the organization Men Can Stop Rape has developed a campaign called My Strength is Not for Hurting and engaged local sports figures to speak out against violence toward women. These examples confirm that it is possible to question such violence and possibly reduce it, even in settings where it is ubiquitous or banal.

Becoming fathers

A key question that has driven much of the research on men's roles in families is whether men as fathers matter in the lives of women and children. In many parts of the world, some women's rights advocates have asked: why devote resources, research and programme efforts, to men's roles as fathers, if after all it is women who provide most of the child care? In the area of child development, many researchers have asked whether in fact children need fathers to develop well. Taken as a whole, the research on fathers and fatherhood affirms that men's participation as fathers, as co-parents and as partners with women in domestic chores, child care and childrearing, does matter, in terms of child well-being, family income, greater equality in the division of household labour and for men themselves.[2]

What does fatherhood mean to young men and how do they react to it? Many young men in poorer countries become fathers in their early to mid-twenties. This act represents, for many, a major role transition, a significant new relationship in their lives and a new social function. Much of the research and discourse about young fathers in low-income settings is negative or relies on negative stereotypes. Young fathers are often presumed to be negligent, irresponsible and seeking to shrug their involvement. But does the reality match these stereotypes?

Several studies suggest that young fathers, like young mothers, may face social pressures to drop out of school to support their children and are less likely to complete secondary school than their non-parenting peers (Barker 2000). Research suggests that many young men may initially deny responsibility and paternity when faced with a possible pregnancy, in large part because of the financial burden associated with caring for a child. For example, research in Mexico suggests that a young father's employment and financial situation were the important factors in determining how the young men reacted to pregnancy and fatherhood (Atkin and Alatorre 1991). Young men with stable employment or more income were more likely to participate in child care and in providing financially for the child.

Young fathers often face stereotypes on the part of their parents, the parents of their child's mother, the mother herself, and service providers. Young fathers who do not marry the mothers of the children, for example, are frequently seen as being irresponsible. However, research finds that in some cases, young fathers may want to be involved with their child, but the child's mother will not allow that involvement unless they are also providing financially for the child. Young fathers who are unemployed may feel constrained in their parenting role because they do not believe they have the right to interact with their child if they are not financially providing for him or her. Such nuances have not been widely studied and are often neglected in discussions about young fathers (Lyra 1998). Indeed, only since around the 1990s have a handful of programmes in several parts of the world started to examine the multiple roles of fathers, and to promote greater involvement by fathers in child care and maternal health.

Many of these initiatives started by listening to the voices of fathers themselves. It is surprising, even disturbing, to see how much of the literature or research on young fathers and fathers in general is told by others – mothers, health care staff, children. Perhaps only since the mid-1980s have researchers and programme staff asked young men themselves about their experiences and challenges. Indeed, when asked about it, young men can be quite articulate about the challenges of fatherhood, relationships and work, as was this young man in Chicago:

> A lot of guys just leave, they disclaim them [their children] . . . You can find a good handful these days [of men who assume responsibility for their children] . . . only a handful of men take care of their children. Most guys leave because they can't deal with the pressure. It's not the fact that he got the female pregnant, but he's also young and he's tryin' to figure out how he's gonna take care of this shorty [baby]. He may be too young to get a job so there's only one other alternative for him to make some money [gangs]. That's enough on his back already, let alone havin' to explain to his parents how this female is havin' his baby. You see all these talk shows with women talkin' about men who don't help . . . Instead of gettin' on the man's back you need to see the pressure they face. You find girls trappin' males . . . they think if they have a child, the man will be with them for life.
>
> (Marty, 18, African American, Chicago)

Other young men, as we have already seen, experience pressure from their families or peers to prove their fertility. Said one young man: 'All my homeys [friends] got kids and I'm the only one who don't have one and they say to me: "Hey, ain't it your time?"'

If much of the discourse about early childbearing – among young women and men – has focused on the negative consequences, there are positive sides to be considered. For some young men, fatherhood is a powerful and positive role transition and an opportunity for organizing their lives. Some young men are able to leave gangs because of fatherhood and describe their child as their 'life cause'. Said one gang-involved young father: 'My daughter just pulls at my heart . . . she makes me want to change. She pulls me up. I feel like my daughter is my purpose to live. I want to be able to give her more' (Juanito, 19, Hispanic, gang-involved, non-custodial father, Chicago).

Said another young father:

> She's [pointing to his daughter] the main reason [I got out of gangs]. I didn't really want this to happen [to be a father] but when she was born I made a promise to myself that I don't want her to go through what I did.
>
> (Kique, 22, Hispanic, formerly gang-involved father, Chicago)

For some young men in Brazil, being a father meant taking whatever kind of work they could find, even those jobs that were considered humiliating or low-paying by some of the other young men (selling candy or other products on the bus or on street corners, guarding parked cars):

> Before I had my daughter, I only knew how to play. The money I was able to make was just for me, like for my house and for my clothes. Now that I have a daughter, my obligation is to her ... if there's anything missing at home, I have to go after it.
>
> (João, 19, young father, Rio de Janeiro).

Some young men describe fatherhood as giving them a sense of connection and a purpose for living. Those individuals who have worked with young fathers and seen them achieve their potential for caregiving and solidarity are frequently awed by the transition.

Conclusions

It is possible, of course, to make a list of young men's commonly perceived deficiencies in relation to their partners and their children, ranging from not providing child support, to limited involvement in domestic chores, to the use of violence against women. As we have seen here, however, these weaknesses are only one part of the story.

Many young men, for example, do not use violence against partners. Similarly, some young men, even from early ages, show a clear preference for more intimate relationships rather than occasional or casual ones. Some boys and girls in diverse cultural settings also experience caregiving in diverse ways from their fathers – which is a tremendous impetus for seeing the world through a different lens, particularly one in which men can also provide caregiving.

These examples and voices of young men suggest that we need to work with them to instil a critical pedagogy – a critical reflection – about what it means to be young men, and about their roles in relationships and as potential or future fathers or father figures. Young men who have used violence against women are generally not happy or content with their use of violence. If given the opportunity to discuss the issue, they often come to realize that a relationship based on fear and violence is not much of a relationship after all. Similarly, those young men who are not involved in the lives of their children are frequently frustrated by the situation and desire some connection with them.

This is all to say that there is a generation of young men out there, waiting for places and ways to think about relationships with women and fatherhood in alternative ways. Changing deeply embedded ideas about gender roles is a formidable challenge, but we see in the voices of some young men presented here that caring, democratic versions of manhood are possible, even in the most traditional of places.

Chapter 10

Dying to be men, living as men

Conclusions and final reflections

What does a gender perspective – and more specifically a focus on young men and masculinities – suggest for preventing violence and promoting greater gender equality and a masculine ethic of care? From the examples presented so far, one of the first and obvious conclusions is that of engaging those young and older men, who already exist in such settings, who show resistance to some of the violent and rigid versions of manhood they see around them.

Indeed, a constant theme in this book has been the variation in the stories and lives of young men. The reductionist and essentialist view that 'men are from Mars, and women are from Venus', or 'that boys will be boys' does not hold up in the face of the variety of young men, women and their realities. This we know: far too many are dying to be men – from violence, from HIV/AIDS, from traffic accidents, from causes that have little to do with genetics or biology and almost everything to do with how boys are socialized. Far too many men behave in ways that are harmful to their own health and that of their partners. But there are always exceptions and there is always potential for change. It is these exceptions that provide a point of entry globally for the purposeful promotion of change in rigid gender orders.

There are always voices of resistance – young men who are able to see through the gender matrix for what it is: a flimsy, sometimes harmful way to organize the world and their personal lives. These young men who 'resist' these rigid or violent versions of manhood often like being boys or men in some traditional ways, such as participating in sports, but they question the notions that women deserve to be beaten, or that caring for children is the work of women, or that a man must fight if he is insulted. It is important to listen to these voices, and to seek to understand what factors make it possible for young men to become respectful, non-violent and caring in their interpersonal relationships.

Understanding resistance and difference

What makes resistance to rigid views about gender possible? Where do voices of equality, respect and non-violence come from, particularly in settings where violence and rigid views about manhood prevail? In listening to young men and interacting with others who know them – parents, girlfriends, wives, teachers and the like – a number of factors emerge.

One is having family members or other influential individuals who modelled or presented alternative, more equitable and non-violent views about gender roles to the young man. This might be a father, an uncle, a teacher, a pastor or priest or imam, or a mother or grandmother, who suggested that other ways of being women and men are possible. A working mother who took on roles often attributed to fathers or men, or a father or uncle who was involved early on in the care of his children, sends powerful messages to sons and daughters about the fluidity of gender roles.

Another factor is having experienced some personal pain or loss as a result of traditional or violent versions of masculinity and having been able to reflect about this loss. This includes a young man who is able to perceive the struggles that his family faced when a father abandoned the family or used violence against the mother. This perception also includes coming to see traditional versions of manhood as having a high personal 'cost'. An example here is provided by one young man in Rio de Janeiro who had seen three men in his family die (from homicide and alcohol-related accidents and health problems) and as a result began to question what it means to be a man. Other examples include young men who have seen brothers, cousins or other persons close to them participate in drug trafficking and have seen the consequences.

With the right support or in the right circumstances, some young men are able to admit or come to see that the exaggerated version of manhood they are trying to live up to is a sham. One young man in Chicago said he had previously been a 'Romeo' – a young man known for his sexual conquests. But over time, he came to see that such behaviour was shallow and self-defeating, and caused him to lose relationships with women he valued:

GB: So you tried to be a Romeo?

LEMAR: Yeah, but it's too much work.

GB: What do you mean too much work?

LEMAR: It's just like you always trying to hide one from the other so they don't find out about each other.

GB: What do your friends who are Romeos feel about your serious relationship?

LEMAR: They just be like: 'I don't see how you can do it [be with just one girl].'

For most young men who resist rigid notions of manhood, it is generally also essential that they found a group of peers, young men like themselves, who also question traditional views about manhood or at the very least, do not criticize or ridicule a young man when he suggests that there is nothing wrong with being gay, that women do not 'deserve' to be beaten or that it is acceptable for a man to express and acknowledge fear. Indeed, few young men are able to achieve gender equity or non-violence in settings where gender-inequitable views and violent versions of manhood hold sway without the help of someone else, or without others who supported their opposition to such views.

For some young men, in settings where gang involvement was common and where gangs are the most visible standard-bearers of manhood, it is important to have another identity, or another 'hat'. Some young men are able to stay out of gangs and question the version of manhood that gangs promoted because they excel in sports, or music or have some culturally relevant skill that allows them to feel secure in achieving a non-violent and more gender-equitable version of manhood. Young men with strong religious convictions – and who found a sense of identity in their religion and a peer group with fellow members of the same religion – are also able to stay out of gangs with relative ease. They have clearly marked their masculinity as non-violent and gangs generally left them alone. For some young men, having a skill – for example, being good with computers, excelling in one or more academic subjects, being involved in a meaningful extra-curricular activity or having mechanical abilities – is a source of belonging, pride and self-esteem, which again, gives them additional personal energy to stay out of gangs. For a few young men, being connected to and finding school to be a safe and welcoming space, is an important reason to stay away from gangs.

In most of the contexts described in this book, there are two key aspects of male identity and two distinct but overlapping pressures. One is to adhere to a version of manhood that promotes the superiority of men over women, the non-involvement of men in sexual and reproductive health issues, the acceptance of violence against women and limited involvement by men in caring for children. At the same time, there is often a pressure to adhere to a violent version of manhood associated with gang involvement, or at least to support the gang-involved version of manhood that encourages the use of violence. Different factors sometimes apply in terms of how young men are able to 'resist', but there are many commonalities.

Many young men who resist are able to try on or rehearse a non-violent or gender-equitable version of manhood and perceived benefits or positive reinforcement from this alternative version of manhood, in effect creating a feedback loop. For example, one young man in Chicago said:

GB: How do you think your friends treat girls?

TAMIR: When I look at them [how other guys treat girls] it kind [*sic*] of make me ashamed . . . Sometimes I want to cry for girls . . . the way they [the guys] treat their girls and how they cheat on them and then you don't understand why the girls stay. They embarrass them in front of everybody and make them look stupid.

GB: And what about you and your friends?

TAMIR: When we hang out together in a group [of young men who respect women], people look at us, especially the girls, and the reputation we put out is the reputation we get. We don't walk around being rude to or disrespecting girls so we kind of get that respect back.

For a few young men, knowledge matters, for example, knowledge about how to care for young children, or where to acquire sexual and reproductive health services. One young man in Chicago had experience caring for his younger siblings. His mother spent time away caring for an ill aunt, and he cared for all the children in his household, changing nappies and the like. His mother insisted that this was good for him, and would be useful when he formed his own family. Over time, he seemed to come to agree with her.

In nearly all of these cases, achieving alternative male identities or ways of being a man required self-reflective abilities – that is living a reflective life – in other words, thinking about the question posed in Chapter 1: 'How did I get to be the man that I am?' Achieving alternative views about manhood involves first and foremost being able to question traditional views about manhood. Younger boys who are trying desperately to fit in, to be socially recognized and not to be seen as 'geeks' or 'wimps' often have tremendous difficulty stepping back and questioning the versions of manhood that are forced upon them. The social pressure is high to be part of certain hegemonic versions of manhood – to fight for your honour, to dominate women and to suppress fear. It is an act of courage in many cases and of tremendous reflection to step away from these contests of traditional manhood and find other ways of being a man.

Most non-violent young men are able to construct a consistent life story that they present to themselves and to their peers, have the ability to make meaning and find lessons out of personal tragedy and have the ability to step back and reflect about who they are. They are, in summary, able to make connections from the disparate events in their lives and draw relevant lessons and conclusions from these experiences, particularly from difficult life moments related to prevailing versions of manhood. Chuckie, a successful student, in talking about a time when he was 10–11 and getting in trouble at school for fighting (also a time he was in a gang), said:

I thought about it and I realized it wasn't worth it. It wasn't worth me failing. It wasn't worth my education and if I keep acting like this somebody gonna hurt me too. If not I'm gonna end up in jail for hurtin' somebody or I'm gonna get kicked out of school . . . and I'm never gonna make it.

(Chuckie, 18, African American, Chicago)

Armando, a 19-year-old Hispanic father struggling to be a non-violent partner and an involved father, when asked how he found a way to be non-violent toward his wife, after having hit her once before, said:

GB: Where do you think you learned how to be a man?

ARMANDO: The truth, I think I'm learning on my own. If I had taken my father's example, I'd have learned to yell at women. After everything I saw in my family, I try to be different. I saw suffering . . . I saw my mother and father crying. There were blows between them. All these things made me want to be different. There was infidelity. I don't want to be that way.

Most of these young men show some degree of metacognition, that is they are able to think about how they think. They also showed a high degree of awareness of their own emotional life, what Howard Gardner (1983) and others have called emotional intelligence. They were able to see when they were losing control, and are able to identify and use coping or anger management strategies. In addition to having coping and anger management abilities, they were aware of when they need to use those strategies. When talking about how they deal with problems, conflicts and moments when they think they might physically harm a young woman, or get into a fight with another man, nearly all these young men can describe some combination of coping or anger control strategies. For some, this involves walking away or leaving the scene; others mention smoking a cigarette, praying, listening to music or walking. Here, it is not only the walking away or listening to music that is important, but also the self-awareness that this strategy works in reducing violence and knowing when to use it.

An important finding of the work and studies presented in this book is that there are multiple and qualitatively different pathways to non-violent and gender-equitable masculinity. For many young men, a decision not to be gang-involved seems to be a cognitive one, based on personal reflection and a sense of self-awareness in which they perceived their lives as having continuity, seeing the consequences of past actions and referring in some cases to values or ideals beyond their daily existence. For others, it is the luck of finding an alternative peer group or having family members who can buffer the pressure of gangs. And for some, unplanned fatherhood forces them to reflect about these issues and to take a stand. It is important to recognize the qualitative differences in these pathways to non-violent and more gender-equitable masculine identities – and to work with young men to explore the various pathways to resistance that are available or relevant to them.

The role of women in the making of men

In many cases, heterosexual young men achieved alterative views about manhood with the support of a female partner, a wife or girlfriend. One young man interviewed in Chicago had been involved in gangs, and spent several years in prison for his participation in gang-related violence. He had three children with three different women but he got out of a gang and assumed responsibility for his youngest child only because the mother of the youngest child wanted to have a relationship with him and believed that he could stay out of gangs:

> She [my fiancée] didn't know how to take it [when I was in jail].You know, she stayed with me. She caught me with about 15 different girls visiting me in jail. I owe her a lot of credit. She stuck it out.
>
> (Kique, 22, Hispanic, Chicago)

Her belief that he could be different – that he did not have to remain stuck in a traditional version of manhood – along with his reflections about the direct costs of his violent manhood, were key to changing his views about manhood. We saw a similar example in the life of João in Rio de Janeiro, who became a father when he was 18. Because he had only occasional employment and income, he lived apart from the mother and his child. The mother's family believed that João was irresponsible, and not good for much. But the mother of the child continued to believe in him, and allowed and encouraged him to spend time with their child and gradually convinced her family that his intentions were good.

These are just two examples of the importance of women and partners in reinforcing changes and resistance to traditional or violent versions of manhood together with young men. The key point is that gender roles are constructed and reconstructed – and must be questioned – by both men *and* women. Girls and women can contribute to traditional, harmful versions of manhood, just as boys and men can contribute to traditional, restrictive versions of womanhood.

If we look at the HIV/AIDS epidemic worldwide and the growing number and proportion of women and girls who are affected, or at the issue of gender-based violence, we are compelled to talk about the vulnerability of women. Unfortunately, far too few initiatives, individuals, heads of state (mostly men) and women themselves have understood that women are made vulnerable by the ways that masculinities are constructed – as well as the ways that womanhood is constructed.

Women are made vulnerable to HIV/AIDS largely because of the behaviour of men – because men have money and favours to pay for sex with younger girls from poor families, because men may refuse to use condoms, because men can and do have outside partners, and so on. Changing gender norms and paradigms requires empowering those who are disempowered and helping those who dominate to see the 'costs' of their domination to themselves and those around them.

In addition to HIV/AIDS, there are other issues where more attention needs to be paid to men. In the case of gender-based violence, it is imperative to protect women from such violence and to create and enforce legal structures that do so. But it is equally important to work with boys and men to question versions of manhood that encourage such violence. Many women who have worked as allies and activists on behalf of abused women have difficulties seeing the potential of men for change. Many nurses, social workers and women's rights activists spend their professional lives listening to stories of men behaving in abhorrent ways and assisting women who have suffered as a result. For these women, it is understandably difficult to believe that much good or potential can be found in men, or that men need to be engaged in such issues.

But true and lasting changes in gender norms will be achieved only when it is widely recognized that gender is relational, that it is short-sighted to seek to empower women without engaging men, and that it is difficult if not impossible to change what manhood means without engaging young women.

Promoting resistance

The previous examples of voices of resistance, and the factors associated with that resistance, are largely 'naturally occurring' factors, that is they happened in low-income, urban communities in several parts of the world largely without the existence of specific programmes or initiatives that sought to produce this change – by individuals and families seeking different and better ways to live their personal lives.[1]

What can we learn about this naturally occurring resistance that can be included in social action to purposefully encourage gender equality among men? Since 2000, a consortium of NGOs (see the Appendix for more information about Program H) has been working in several settings in Brazil and Mexico to use this information on voices of resistance to design initiatives to engage young men in promoting greater gender equality. For example, if peer groups are important in supporting different views about manhood, it may be possible to create alternative peer groups for young men that support gender equality.

The participating organizations also developed a community campaign using the media, advertising and youth culture to promote gender equality among young men as being 'cool' or hip. Just as many private sector advertising campaigns seek to promote a lifestyle associated with their product, this campaign uses mass media and youth culture to promote a gender-equitable lifestyle among young men. In Brazil, the campaign has been called Hora H or In the Heat of the Moment. The phrase was developed by young men themselves, who frequently heard their peers say: 'Everybody knows you shouldn't hit your girlfriend, but in the heat of the moment you lose control.' Or, 'Everybody knows that you should use a condom, but in the heat of the moment . . .' Campaign slogans thus use language from the community and images of young men from the same communities acting in ways that support gender equality. One of the slogans says: 'In the heat of the moment, a real man . . . cares, listens, accepts.' Young men themselves designed a graffiti-style logo for the campaign that adorns T-shirts and hats and has become a well-known symbol of gender equality in these communities.

Importantly, this campaign does not directly question gangs or gang violence in the community. Indeed, to speak out openly against the gangs in these settings would be dangerous for the safety of the young men and project staff. But by promoting alternative ways of being a man, the initiative seeks to capture the hearts and minds of young men who might be attracted to gangs or to violent versions of manhood. The campaign billboards are in effect advertisements for a different version of manhood, one based on respect and dialogue rather than violence. The campaign seeks to counter the 'glory' and attention that has been directed toward gang-involved young men.

In addition, if other important individuals are important in encouraging resistance, the initiative has carried out outreach activities in the community to engage adult men and women in discussions about what it means to be a man. Project staff have also engaged more gender-equitable adult men from these same communities to act as mentors or group coordinators.

Given the importance of self-reflective abilities, staff developed and tested a set of group educational activities that focus on promoting reflections about the 'costs' of traditional views about manhood. Group educational activities were field-tested with nearly 300 young men aged 15–24 in six countries in Latin America and the Caribbean (Brazil, Peru, Mexico, Bolivia, Colombia and Jamaica). Qualitative results from field-testing found that participation in the activities led to increased empathy, reduced conflict among participants and positive reflection among participants about how they treated their female partners. One young man who participated in the field test process in Peru said: 'After the activities, we came to see the ways we are *machista* . . . you know, treat women unfairly.' Another young man said: 'I realized how I sometimes became violent, because that's the way I was treated. I saw the connection.' Programme staff have also sought to engage numerous allies in the community in these efforts – ranging from schools to health centres – so that several voices in the same community are promoting alternative views about manhood.

As part of the initiative, an evaluation tool was developed, called the Gender-Equitable Men Scale (GEM Scale), which assesses young men's attitudes related to gender roles and masculinities and is also used to measure changes in attitudes. Working in low-income communities in Rio de Janeiro, the Horizons Program and Instituto Promundo carried out an impact evaluation study. Initial results from two communities, from comparing pre-test and post-test surveys with approximately 450 of the more than 780 young men that were included in the pre-test, found increased condom use with regular partners, decreased rates of self-reported symptoms of sexually transmitted infections and positive change on the great majority of the 17 attitude questions used to assess changes in views about gender.[2]

Project staff have also interviewed a selection of young men before and after the activities, and with young women who are the girlfriends or partners of the young men (Horizons 2004). Many young men told us examples of how the workshops had helped them question views about manhood.

However promising this approach may be, however, 780 young men at a time will not lead to the level of social change required to improve the lives of a substantial portion of the world's young people. As part of efforts to scale-up such activities, the collaborating organizations are working with various international agencies and ministries of health to make these activities part of national HIV/AIDS prevention programmes and initiatives, and part of the public health system at the highest level of policy.

Program H, of course, is not the only programme trying to promote such change. From South Africa, to Nigeria, to India and the Philippines, to parts of Central America, South America and the Caribbean, a growing number of programmes and individuals are doing similar things to encourage young men to question what it means to be a man. These programmes have shown that men can and will change when engaged in appropriate, participatory ways to question traditional views about manhood. Indeed, for many young men, some aspects of traditional manhood turn out to be flimsy shams that are fairly easily unravelled or deconstructed by provoking thoughtful and critical reflection as well as interactions with young men who have come to question traditional gender roles.[3]

Changing behaviour is complex and difficult and requires working at the individual, community and societal level, but it is possible. It also requires bringing about changes in the basic ways that men and women order their worlds. It is not simply about promoting condom use, however important that is. Nor is reducing men's violence against women as simple as teaching anger management techniques like counting to 10 or going for a walk when you are angry. Nor is engaged fatherhood simply teaching young men how to change nappies.

All of these traditional behaviours – violence against women, non-involvement in sexual and reproductive health issues and the like – are rooted in deeply held beliefs. To change the behaviour, it is necessary to work with young men to question these beliefs – to question the gender matrix – at the societal and individual level. Too often, though, groups working with young men merely provide information or become preachy without understanding the motivations and viewpoints of young men. It is long overdue to become more sophisticated about promoting gender equality and non-violence.

The silence of young men in the face of social exclusion

Behind the stories of the young men presented here are challenges, personal loss, frustration and individual pain. By calling attention to the challenges young men face, it is imperative that we do not make them into the new victims of the month. The point is that young men face consequences of living in poverty and social exclusion – and experience this frustration in gender-specific and age-specific ways. However, few of these young men reported having spaces to deal with or process the pain and feelings associated with family-related and personal struggles. Few of the young men spoke of outlets, either individual or group, to express the pain or struggles associated with the litany of issues they faced: abandonment by fathers, domestic violence, alcoholism, death of family members, and/or having been victims of some violence (or witnessed friends or family members be victims).

While the interviews with young men reported in this book were not deliberately therapeutic, merely asking the young men to talk about their life stories offered a space – for many the first time they had that space – to discuss such issues. A common response at the end of the discussions was: 'No one ever asked me about that before' or 'I have never talked about these issues before.'

However, if their lives are characterized by family stresses and personal struggles, these young men should not be portrayed as passive in the face of poverty and social exclusion. The young men displayed an impressive array of survival skills, humour and energy in coping with the ongoing challenges of living in social exclusion. It was common for them to study, work part-time (in the evenings, weekends, and/or during school breaks) and have family-related duties (such as taking care of other family members). In summary, it was easy to come away from the interviews impressed by how diligently these young men were coping and struggling to do the right thing for themselves and their families and partners. Such discourses are vital to highlight given the prevailing negative stereotypes about low-income young men.

Clearly too few young men – and young women – have places where they can express this frustration. This is not to advocate for individual or group therapy for all young men in low-income settings. It is instead to emphasize the need to create cultures of gender and manhood in which young men are encouraged to express their frustration and personal pain in ways that do not include physical violence or substance abuse.

Bright moments in violent places

Listening to men talk about these issues means hearing a young man describe how and why he beat his girlfriend, or listening to another young man describe his participation in a gang rape, or hearing how a young man had been tortured by police (men) and of another who participated in the killing of other young men. Part of the information-gathering or fieldwork for this book has meant seeing men addicted to opium lying in the doorways of brothels, men engaged in drunken brawls, men crying over a child they could not be with and young men unrepentant for having passed on a sexually transmitted infection to their girlfriends. This book could have focused on the harmful and sometimes reprehensible behaviour of young men; there is no shortage of such behaviours and there is ample literature that describes it.

Such stories must be told, but the choice was made to emphasize the other stories – those of resistance and hope. Developmental psychologist Erik Erikson (1969) wrote that hope is the basic component of all change and vitality, of development. To believe that change is possible – that fewer men have to die or kill or injure others to prove their manhood – requires finding hope and bright moments in violent places. This work deliberately set out to find voices of resistance in the midst of men behaving badly.

One example is Anderson, a young men who had been in a gang, and whose family had few men because they had died through violence or alcohol abuse. He had spent time living on the streets, was imprisoned and faced a drug addiction. He was immensely behind in his schooling and had few job prospects. But over the course of three years, he became an engaged father and a spokesperson for a group of young men working with other young men to promote gender equality. Another example is Jeferson, who had witnessed his stepfather beat his mother to the point of suffering hearing loss, and who had used violence against a girl himself. When we began working with him he looked to the ground and seldom spoke up. Over the course of a couple of years, he too went on to become an active member of a group of young men working to promote gender equality and non-violence with other young men. He was completing secondary school and sought to study in university to become a psychologist, saying he wanted to pursue a career in helping others.

Examples were included of young men in Nigeria, who in the face of tremendous gender inequalities, had an almost religious fervour to engage other men in discussions about how to treat women in more respectful ways. In South Africa, we spoke with a support group of HIV-positive men, nearly all fathers, ranging from age 19 to early forties. These men defy the stereotype that men do not generally disclose their HIV status, or that men blame women for HIV. These were men who openly – in groups of men and women – acknowledged their risky sexual behaviour and sought to support their families to the best of their abilities. In Uganda, we interviewed a young man who was HIV-positive. He had become a peer outreach worker with an AIDS prevention programme and met his wife, also HIV-positive, through the programme. With orientation from the organization, they have since had a child, 9 months old, who is HIV-negative:

GB: What do you wish for your son?
EDWARD: God-willing, I will be around to see my son finish his schooling and maybe go on to university . . . who knows, maybe he'll work with TASO [The AIDS Support Organization of Uganda].

In Soweto in South Africa we met young men previously involved in self-defence units affiliated with the ANC, who carried out killings against members of the self-defence units of youth affiliated with the Inthaka Freedom Party (a rival black political party to the ANC during the time of transition to democracy in South Africa). During the final years of the apartheid regime and the transition to democratic rule, the outgoing apartheid government encouraged violent confrontations between the two political groups. The young men we spoke with had since become colleagues or friends with their former Inthaka rivals. Working in partnership with EngenderHealth, they currently engage out-of-school youth in their community to provide job-readiness training and group sessions to question traditional views about gender and manhood. Said one of the founders of the programme:

> The trauma of the early 1990s is still here . . . some young men here saw their parents killed. With the necklacing [killing of rivals by putting a tyre around their neck, filling it with petrol and then burning it], many times the body would be left on the street for a month or more . . . I myself was a soldier with the ANC . . . we didn't know if at any time, the police would come into our house [and arrest us, or kill us]. Nobody understood why we were fighting. It was black against black. We didn't even know what we were dying for. Houses were burnt.
>
> Even up to the elections [in 1994], there was violence . . . and there was silence around this violence. There were no police around [in 1994] in those days, everyone carried guns. Parents were not around to parent. Youth were raising themselves. Parents fled to their home states because of the violence. During the violence, you had no money . . . so you would go for crime for money. Your parents weren't around . . .

> Now we offer life skills and HIV/AIDS activities. When we found them [the youth currently involved in their project], they were bored, doing nothing ... we try to get them life skills ... that helps them develop a goal and a vision. We're trying to help them change their mindset, to get over their violent past.

This is the hope that sustains voices of resistance and helps restore dignity to being a young man. It should not be shameful to be a young man living in a low-income setting. No young man should be treated as a walking deficit or potential criminal, or sexual predator in the making. Even after men have acted in ways that are harmful to themselves, or their partners or others around them, we must still, as Erikson (1996) suggested, look for the hope that sustains positive change and development.

For too long, the violent young men and the reprehensible behaviour of some young men have earned the headlines and attention, and when they have, it has generally been to demonize them rather than to understand how such behaviour emerges. The young men described in this book represent stories of mostly unrecognized and quiet dignity, courage, caring and positive coping – voices of peace and resistance that are generally overshadowed by the kind of masculinity promoted by gangs. Violent young men, particularly those in gangs, succeed in getting noticed. They attract young women. They cause unease among their peers and neighbours by their use of violence. They get headlines and frighten the middle class. Many die in dramatic gunfights with rival gangs or with police. They are the subjects of seminars, dissertations, movies and documentaries.

But the voices of resistance are mostly in the shadows. Their stories should be the headlines, but just as João said that the gangbangers get the girls, tragedy and violence generally make more appealing headlines and move policy-makers to action, usually in counterproductive ways. By listening to the voices of resistance, by engaging them in programme efforts and policy development, it is possible to resist rigid and violent versions of manhood and in the process to help more young men achieve a masculine ethic of care, respect and empathy.

Background on research sites and methodology

The interviews and interactions with young men reported in this book emerge from several different research projects from 1994 to 2004. The following is a brief overview of these research sites, the methodology and some of the major findings.

Caribbean, 1994–95

The interviews with young men in the Caribbean were carried out as part of a needs assessment on substance use, drug trafficking and low-income youth (the vast majority young men), carried out for the United Nations Office on Drugs and Crime (UNODC, formerly UNDCP). The following methodologies were used:

- focus group discussions and small group discussions with at-risk young people
- interviews with key informants, including government officials, staff of governmental and non-governmental organizations assisting youth, and community leaders or other individuals with direct access to at-risk young people
- direct observation and interaction with at-risk young people.

Interviews were carried out in St Vincent and the Grenadines, Trinidad and Tobago, St Maarten and Jamaica. Jamaica and Trinidad and Tobago were chosen because they are the two most populous countries in the English-speaking Caribbean and have the largest concentrations of urban poverty, and hence the largest populations of low-income young people. St Maarten and St Vincent were chosen as being representative of smaller English-speaking Caribbean islands which have emerging problems of substance use and drug trafficking among young men. More than thirty focus groups were carried out in total, along with nearly sixty interviews with key informants. Interviews and interactions with young men took place in schools, youth centres, mental institutions, prisons and in rural communities. The final report is included in Barker et al. (1995).

Chicago, 1997–98

Data from Chicago came from two different studies, one with younger boys (aged 11–14) and one with older boys and young men (aged 15–20). The study with younger boys included focus group discussions and individual interviews with twenty-three boys (aged 11–14) who were participating in sexuality education programmes at two public schools, one mostly Hispanic and the other mostly African American. This included limited interaction with students and staff who carried out the sexuality education programme.

Young men participating in the second study included 25 African American and Hispanic young men aged 15–20; six of the young men were fathers. The initial purpose of this study was to carry out a small number of exploratory in-depth individual interviews and focus group discussions with young men who were participating in three different programmes supported by a social service agency in Chicago (the Ounce of Prevention Fund). As the interviews unfolded, two issues became apparent. First, it became clear that the pathways toward gang involvement and other forms of delinquency, violence toward and attitudes toward women, and attitudes related to fatherhood, were intertwined. Second, it became clear that the young men who were attracted to participate in the activities run by the social service agency – a 'male responsibility discussion group' at one site, and a teen fathers' discussion group in the other site – were, not surprisingly, different to the typical young men in their neighbourhoods in terms of being more pro-social, progressive and non-violent. Thus in seeking to understand the young men who were participating in this social service agency's activities, we found ourselves studying pro-social and non-violent males. Therefore, the research evolved into a preliminary qualitative exploration of the factors associated with being pro-social and non-violent in settings where the prevailing models of masculinity are those that promote gang involvement, delinquency, uninvolved fathering and negative attitudes toward women.

The qualitative methodologies used were:

- in-depth individual interviews
- focus group discussions
- participant observation with the males in a school setting and in a social service agency.

These qualitative research methods were used as an exploratory tool to begin identifying possible variables or factors associated with being a non-violent male in violent communities.

Being a 'non-violent and pro-social male' was defined as:

- not being gang-involved at the time of the interview, were currently seeking to leave a gang or were not involved in other forms of delinquency;
- demonstrated values of respect toward women and repudiated violence toward women
- believed that males should take responsibility for their children and hoped to be, or actively sought to be, involved fathers.

To be sure, not all the young men interviewed fit this definition of non-violent and pro-social equally well. Some seemed firmly anchored in a violent male identity, while others were still struggling with such issues. Nonetheless as a starting point for discussion, this definition was useful.

The bulk of the interviews took place during a four-month period of time, with interactions in the social service agency and school ranging over more than nine months. Access to these two groups of young men was facilitated by staff at both sites. All young men participating were volunteers, and for all subjects, signed informed consent was obtained.

In addition to this formal study, I also spent one afternoon a week in the public high school where the 'male responsibility' group was carried out. For these sessions, extensive field notes were gathered. Both studies were supported in part by the Ounce of Prevention Fund (for whom the research provided insights for engaging young men in existing programmes), the Chapin Hall Center for Children at the University of Chicago and the Open Society Institute. Portions of this study were published in Barker (1998).

Rio de Janeiro, 1994–95

This study included focus group discussions with 127 adolescents and young adults, aged 14–30, men and women, in two vocational training programmes for low-income young people. About half of the interviewees were young women, although the emphasis was on young men. The comments of young women were mostly used as triangulation, or seeking their opinions on the attitudes and behaviour of men.

Respondents were divided into two age ranges (14–18 and 19–30) to attempt to understand how the construction of gender differed over these two cohorts. Focus groups were homogenous; groups were chosen from existing classrooms in which youth were grouped according to grade and age.

In each focus group, there were one or two young men who questioned the prevailing views that sex for men is seen as an uncontrollable urge, that violence against women was justifiable in cases of infidelity and the general lack of male involvement in reproductive health issues. Subsequently, eight individual interviews were carried out with these more gender-equitable young men, nearly all of whom reported and described in detail relationships or interactions with a relative or friend who modelled or supported non-traditional gender roles. This study is presented in Barker and Loewenstein (1997).

Rio de Janeiro, 1999–2001

Building on the 1994–95 study, and on the research in Chicago, in 1999, a two-year qualitative research project was commenced with a group of young men acting in ways that are more gender-equitable than the prevailing norms in the community. The two questions that oriented this study are:

- How are these more gender-equitable young men different than their less gender-equitable peers?
- What can we learn from their lives that might offer insights on how to encourage gender-equitable attitudes and behaviours among other young men?

Health outreach workers, teachers and community-based organizations were asked to help identify a group or individual young men who were 'more gender-equitable'. This term was initially loosely defined to refer to young men who were involved fathers, or showed some interest in health issues (and sought health services), and/or were known as treating their female partners well or with respect. The study concentrated mostly on non-gang-involved young men. Thus, the study sought to identify factors associated with staying out of gangs and factors associated with being more gender-equitable.

Over the course of the study, in interviewing young men, the concept of 'gender-equitable' young men was operationalized to refer to the following:

- Young men who are respectful in their relationships with young women and currently seek relationships based on equality and intimacy rather than sexual conquest and believe that men and women have equal rights, and that women have as much sexual desire and 'right' to sexual agency as do men.
- Young men who seek to be involved fathers, for those who are already fathers, meaning that they believe that they should take financial and at least some caregiving responsibility for their children. They have shown this involvement by providing at least some child care, showing concern for providing financially for the child, and/or take an active role in caring for their child's health.
- Young men who assume some responsibility for reproductive health issues. This includes taking the initiative to discuss reproductive health

concerns with their partner, using condoms or assisting their partner in acquiring or using a contraceptive method.

- Young men who do not use violence against women in their intimate relationships, and are opposed to violence against women. This may include young men who report having been violent toward a female partner in the past, but who currently believe that violence against women is not acceptable behaviour, and who do not condone this behaviour by other men.

These four criteria for 'gender-equitable' should be considered exploratory. They are based in part on what have been the stated goals of male involvement in sexual and reproductive health projects, and in part on what women say they want from men. Using these four criteria, a more detailed, exploratory rating scale was devised to rank the young men as high, medium or low on gender equity. The young men were then ranked using field notes and interview transcripts. The ranking scales focused on behaviours and attitudes with more weight given to the young men's reported behaviour. Interviews with family members, staff who work with the young men and personal observation were also used to assess the young men's degree of gender-equitability. A second reader read the interview transcripts of some of the young men to provide an independent ranking of the young men, which was consistent with my ratings in more than 80 per cent of cases.

Few if any of the young men interviewed achieved all four of these characteristics all the time, if ever. Nonetheless, the research identified an important minority of young men who at least part of the time demonstrated a higher degree of gender-equitable behaviour and attitudes in their interactions with young women than did most of their peers and adult men in the same setting. For most of the young men, it is more appropriate to consider them to be in transition in terms of gender roles rather than truly gender-equitable. While some of the young men interviewed reported having had sexual relationships with other men, all of the young men identified themselves as heterosexual, and the research focused on their intimate relationships with women.

Research methods included observation and interaction with twenty-five young men aged 15–21 two days a week for one year; three formal focus group discussions and approximately fifteen informal group discussions with young men, young women and adults in the community; a three-part life history interview with nine of these young men; interviews with four family members who were willing to be interviewed; and approximately fifteen key informant interviews in the community.

Because the definitions of gender-equitable were being developed as the research progressed (and because we were also developing interventions for work with young men while study was going on), the research was an iterative, ethnographically oriented qualitative study. Over the course of the first two years of the study, I was able to observe major life changes and events, including accompanying the young men during the formation and dissolution of relationships, pregnancies (some terminated, some carried to term), entering the military or acquiring employment, and numerous individual crises and triumphs.

The twenty-five young men who form the larger group from which nine were chosen for individual interviews represent a self-selected group of young men in the community who were participating in a young men's discussion group on health and sexuality. From this group of twenty-five, who are already slightly different in terms of gender norms by participating in the discussion group, we asked the group leaders to identify a number of young men who showed at least one or two of the criteria for being more 'gender-equitable' as described above, and/or had a fairly significant history of relationships with young women (i.e. they had a relationship history to talk about in an interview setting). Nearly all of the young men in the larger group of 25 met these two criteria. Final selection of the nine young men within this group thus was partly convenience sampling, with a bias toward the young men who were slightly older (17 and up) because they had more life history to relate.

Most of the twenty-five young men who had been participating in a young men's discussion group represent a group of young men who are not involved in the *comandos* (although many have brothers or other family members who are), not succeeding in school and generally not working full-time – young men who seem in some ways to lack a place to fit. Some of the young men stood out in the community for the fact that they are vocal and visible – composing rap songs that promote peace instead of violence. The young men, while not involved with *comandos*, report that they have good relationships with the *comando*; indeed, it is dangerous to speak out openly against the *comando*.

The young men interviewed were almost all classmates, neighbours or friends. Nearly all characterize themselves as black or 'Afro', referring to 'Afro-brasileiro'. Nearly all of these young men were studying at the primary level (up until eighth grade), and thus are generally several years behind their age-grade level; most have had less than five years of formal education.

Analysis of transcribed interviews and group discussions focused on identifying factors at three levels – the individual level, the family level and the wider social context – that seem to have enabled these young men to acquire a more gender-equitable male identity than the prevailing norms, and to stay out of gangs.

Since completing the formal portion of the research, involvement has been maintained with many of the young men, some of whom went on to become peer promoters or outreach workers, to engage other young men, at Instituto Promundo. As such, it has been possible to continue to observe and interact with the young men as they have assumed leadership positions beyond their communities. Indeed, one of the main strategies at Instituto Promundo has been to engage as many gender-equitable young men as possible to be outreach workers to promote gender equality among their peers.

This study was funded by the Open Society Institute, and portions were published in Barker (2000b).

Program H, the Gender-Equitable Men Scale, and the Impact Evaluation Study, Brazil, 2000–04

These examples and voices of resistance from our previous studies in Chicago and in Brazil, combined with our direct experience working with men in various parts of the Americas region, led to the formation of Program H – Engaging Young Men in the Promotion of Health and Gender Equity. The initiative was developed in 1999 by four Latin American NGOs that had significant experience in working with young men: Instituto Promundo (coordinator of the initiative, based in Rio de Janeiro, Brazil), ECOS-Communiçacão em Sexualidade (in São Paulo, Brazil), Instituto PAPAI (Recife, Brazil) and Salud y Género (Mexico).

Program H focuses on helping young men question traditional norms related to manhood. It consists of four components:

- a field-tested curriculum that includes a manual series and an educational video for promoting attitude and behaviour change among men
- a lifestyle social marketing campaign for promoting changes in community or social norms related to what it means to be a man
- a research-action methodology for reducing barriers to young men's use of health services
- a culturally relevant validated evaluation tool (the GEM Scale) for measuring changes in attitudes and social norms around manhood.

These components were developed in large part based on the baseline research, previously mentioned, which identified important programmatic implications: first, the need to offer young men opportunities to interact with gender-equitable role models in their own community setting, and second, the need to promote more gender-equitable attitudes in small group settings and in the greater community. This previous research confirmed the need to intervene not only at the level of individual attitude and behaviour change, but also at the level of social or community norms, including among parents, service providers and others that influence these individual attitudes and behaviours.

The activities in the manual series are designed to be carried out in a same-sex group setting, and generally with men as facilitators who also serve as more gender-equitable role models for the young men. The activities consist of role plays, brainstorming exercises, discussion sessions and individual reflections about how boys and men are socialized, positive and negative aspects of this socialization, and the benefits of changing certain behaviours. The themes in the manuals were selected based on a review of literature on the health and development of boys, and an international survey of programmes working with young men. First and foremost, the activities in the manuals and the group educational process focus on creating a safe space to allow young men to question traditional views about manhood.

The activities in the manuals reinforce each other and make appropriate links between specific activities and themes. The manuals are printed in Portuguese, Spanish and English, and are currently widely used in Latin America by NGOs and by ministries of health. The themes of the manuals are:

- sexual and reproductive health
- violence and violence prevention (including gender-based violence prevention)
- reasons and emotions, which focuses on mental health issues and young men, particularly communication skills, dialogue, emotional intelligence and substance use
- fatherhood and caregiving, which encourages young men to reconsider their roles in caregiving in the family, including caring for children
- HIV/AIDS, including both prevention and caregiving.

The manuals are accompanied by a no-words cartoon video, called *Once Upon a Boy*, which presents the story of a young man from early childhood through adolescence to early adulthood. Scenes include the young man witnessing violence in his home, interactions with his male peer group, social pressures to behave in certain ways to be seen as a 'real man', his first unprotected sexual experience, having a sexually transmitted infection and facing an unplanned pregnancy. The video was developed in workshop processes with young men in diverse settings in Latin America and the Caribbean.

In addition to the Program H curriculum, Promundo, JohnSnowBrazil and SSL International (makers of Durex condoms) developed a 'lifestyle social marketing' process for promoting a more gender-equitable lifestyle among men in a given cultural setting. This involves working with men themselves to identify their preferred sources of information, identify young men's cultural outlets in the community and craft messages – in the form of radio spots, billboards, posters, postcards and dances – to make it 'cool and hip' to be a more 'gender-equitable' man. This campaign encourages young men to reflect about how they act as men and enjoins them to respect their partners, not to use violence against women and to practise safer sex. Several major rap artists have been engaged in Brazil to endorse the campaign – which they have called a 'campaign against machismo' – and have presented it during various concerts in Brasilia and Rio de Janeiro.

The campaign taps into youth culture – music, theatre and a knowledge of where young people hang out – to promote more gender-equitable versions of manhood. As described in Chapter 10, this lifestyle social marketing component uses mass media and youth culture to promote a gender-equitable lifestyle among young men. Campaign slogans use language from the community and images are of young men from the same communities – acting in ways that support gender equality.

In 2002, the Program H collaborating organizations began a two-year impact evaluation study. The main impact evaluation tool was the GEM Scale. A list of 35 attitude questions was originally developed related to:

- gender roles in the home and child caregiving
- gender roles in sexual relationships
- shared responsibility for reproductive health and disease prevention
- intimate partner violence
- homosexuality and close relationships with other men.

Attitude questions or statements included affirmations of traditional gender norms, such as: 'Men are always ready to have sex.' 'A woman's most important role is to take care of her home and cook for her family.' 'There are times when a woman deserves to be beaten.' They also included affirmations of more gender-equitable views, such as: 'A man and a woman should decide together what type of contraceptive to use.' 'It is important that a father is present in the lives of his children, even if he is no longer with the mother.' These attitude questions were crafted based on the definition of gender-equitable that was developed, as well as a review of the literature on gender norms and socialization among young men (Barker 2003).

The attitude questions were tested in a community-based survey, and data from this sample were used to test the usefulness of the items and create the final scale. The final scale has twenty-four items. For each item, three answer choices were provided: I agree, I partially agree, and I do not agree. The baseline study was carried out in three communities in Rio de Janeiro, two of which were low-income areas and one of which was a middle-income neighbourhood. In this testing of the GEM Scale, the research team applied a questionnaire to a total of 749 men aged 15–60. All interviewers were male. The questionnaire was administered via a household survey to a random sample of men in each of the three neighbourhoods. The refusal rate was less than 2 per cent.

Baseline testing of the GEM Scale confirmed that the attitude questions held together, meaning that young men answered in fairly internally consistent ways. That is, a young man who said he tolerated or even supported violence against women was also likely to show traditional or male-dominant views on other questions, such as believing that taking care of children was exclusively a woman's responsibility. In addition, the ways young men answered the questions were correlated to how they say they act. In sum, our baseline research confirmed that the GEM Scale is a useful tool for assessing where men are on these issues, or to assess their current attitudes about gender roles, and is also useful for measuring whether they changed their attitudes over time, or after a given project. Young men's attitudes were highly correlated with one of our key outcomes: self-reported use of violence against women. The resulting scale was deemed sufficiently reliable (alpha > 0.80) for use as an evaluation instrument.

With the GEM Scale validated, in 2002, Instituto Promundo and the Horizons Program started a two-year impact evaluation study to measure the impact of different components of Program H, including the manuals and video, and the 'lifestyle' social marketing campaign. The evaluation was done with a sample of approximately 750 young men aged 15–24 in Rio de Janeiro. The study included three different groups of young men in different (but fairly homogeneous) low-income communities (although due to violence in one of the communities, the follow-up sample size was small). With each group of young men, various levels of intensities of the activities were carried out (14 hours of activities in one group, 28 hours of activities in another, and group activities combined with an intense lifestyle social marketing campaign in a third). In one of the communities, the intervention was delayed with the evaluation questionnaire being carried out twice before any intervention is carried out. Utilizing this study design increases the probability that any attitude or behaviour change measured in the intervention groups is the result of the intervention as opposed to other factors.

The young men participating in the study typically engage in a number of risky sexual behaviours. At baseline, more than 70 per cent of the young men were sexually active, with an average age of 13 for sexual initiation. Of the sexually active group, 30 per cent reported more than one sexual partner over the last month. Approximately 25 per cent of the young men reported STI symptoms during the three months prior to the survey. About 10 per cent of young men reported using sexual or physical violence against their current or most recent regular partner.

Fewer than two-thirds (63 per cent) reported condom use at last sex with a primary partner, and 85 per cent reported condom use at last sex with a secondary partner. However, consistent condom use during the last month was higher among men with their regular partners. For young men with casual partners, they were less likely to report consistent condom use with every casual partner over the last month.

At baseline, inequitable gender norms and attitudes were significantly associated with HIV risk. Agreement with more traditional gender roles was significantly associated reported STI symptoms (p < 0.05), lack of contraceptive use (p = 0.05), and physical or sexual violence against a current or recent partner (p < 0.001). Preliminary post-intervention results gathered at six months revealed positive changes at both intervention sites, including significant positive changes in gender norms (Horizons 2004).

At both sites, reported STI symptoms decreased and condom use at last sex with a primary partner increased, and in Bangu, the site where group educational activities were combined with the lifestyle social marketing component, the improvements were statistically significant. The percentage of informants at both sites who reported having two or more partners also decreased somewhat, but not significantly. It was not necessarily more intensity that led to the higher degree of change, but likely the combination of the two intervention components that led to the higher difference.

Findings suggest that educational interventions for young men can successfully influence their attitudes toward gender roles and provide empirical evidence that a behaviour change intervention focused on gender dynamics can lead to reduced HIV/STI risk. They also highlight the importance of reinforcing gender-equity messages on the community level.

Kaduna and Calabar, Nigeria, 2003

The interviews with men in Nigeria were part of a study for the World Bank on young men at-risk within a gender perspective, with a specific focus on violence and conflict (and protective factors that reduce violence) and behaviours and attitudes related to HIV/AIDS. The study includes:

- an in-depth conceptual piece and analytic literature review on young men at-risk from a gender perspective, with a focus on violence and conflict prevention and resolution, including the specific realities and needs of young men in countries emerging from conflict
- an in-depth conceptual piece and analytic literature review on young men at-risk from a gender perspective, with a focus on how the socialization and behaviour of young men contributes to the spread of HIV/AIDS in sub-Saharan Africa
- a review and analysis of promising approaches to engaging young men in reducing violence and promoting safer sex behaviour and gender equity, among young men, with a focus on sub-Saharan Africa.

During fieldwork in Nigeria in November 2003, seven focus group discussions were carried out with young men, ranging in ages from 15 to 40, and met with representatives from twenty organizations, including community-based programmes, government offices and international donors. Limited examples were also included from Uganda and South Africa, which are also included in the study. At the time of completing this book, the data from this study was still being analysed.

Notes

1 Why the worry about young men?

1 Secondary analysis from a 2002 study carried out by Instituto Promundo and Instituto Noos in Brazil (see Instituto Promundo and Instituto Noos 2003).

2 'Are you a hippy or a kicker?'

1 All names of young men used in this book are pseudonyms.
2 In the gender literature, the issue of male circumcision in such conditions has been noticeably absent, focusing mostly on female genital cutting. Of course, the implications and conditions of female genital cutting are different in important ways from the circumcision of male adolescents, and vary by country. Nonetheless, it is noteworthy that similar risks faced by young men are often taken for granted or that our prevailing gender discourse sees socially proscribed genital cutting as a risk for girls and young women, but 'normal' for boys and young men, even when male circumcision in such settings also brings health risks for young men.
3 The information on the male circumcision in the Gisu region of Uganda, while relatively brief here, is based on interviews carried out with young men and adult men in the region in April 2004. An insightful discussion on the issue can be found in Heald (1999).
4 Developmental psychologist Erik Erikson likened adolescent development or identity development to trying on a series of hats before settling on one identity. While this model is sometimes rigid or sometimes interpreted in simplistic ways, it is a useful metaphor for thinking about how individuals achieve a given identity. See, for example, Erikson (1968).
5 The Appendix provides a short overview of the research methodologies and research questions. It also describes a questionnaire and scale – called the Gender-Equitable in Men Scale or GEM Scale – developed together with several colleagues that seeks to assess the degree to which a given sample of young men adhere to more callous/*machista* views about manhood or more gender-equitable versions. The scale serves both as a needs assessment or diagnostic tool – that is for understanding a given population of young men – as well as an evaluation instrument for measuring changes in young men's attitudes on the issues. The instrument is designed to be used in collaboration with qualitative research methodologies, including in-depth individual interviews, observation and focus group discussions. These research projects have been action-research in the sense that they were carried out with the explicit purpose of developing new interventions or refining existing ones.

3 'Don't worry, I'm not a thief'

1 Various ideas and group techniques were developed to keep the group engaged: a talking stick ritual to promote respect for the flow of discussion, outings, holding the sessions in different spaces. Some of these techniques are included in Instituto Promundo et al. (2002).

2 I suggested that we all accompany him and learn where to take our children to be vaccinated and to meet the health post staff. The health post staff were less than thrilled to see a group of 15 young men, most in shorts and sandals, but they accepted us.

3 The process of getting a birth certificate in Brazil is fairly easy, although it requires one of the biological parents to register the child. After turning 18, however, getting a birth certificate requires the action of a judge, something João says he has been trying to do, and with which a colleague of ours provided assistance.

4 The term *Afro-brasileiro* or African Brazilian is gaining use in the media and among some advocacy organizations in Brazil, but is not a term the young men used spontaneously to describe themselves.

5 In early 2000, a number of *favelas* started riots after incidents in which police officers killed residents who were not involved in the *comandos*.

4 The trouble with young men

1 All three neighborhoods had high rates of crime and gang-related crime. The high school in south Chicago is located near a major intersection and public housing project where gang and police shootouts are common. The youth centre where activities and interviews were carried out with young men in one of the Hispanic neighbourhoods is also located in an area of gang activity; on one occasion during the course of the work there, activities at the youth centre were cancelled due to violence between two rival gangs. As of the mid-1990s, Chicago police estimated that 40,000 young people were involved in gangs (Block and Block 1995).

2 In all four settings, there were commonly used negative or stigmatizing expressions used by the middle class to refer to low-income young men, *bandidos, favelas, marginais* in Brazil; rude boys in the Caribbean, hooligans in Nigeria, and so on. In many cases, young men internalized these names and took them as their own.

5 In the headlines

1 By contrast, 33,000 young women aged 15–29 were the victims of homicide worldwide. Homicides of young men aged 15–29 in the Americas represent nearly 14 per cent of the world's annual homicides, although the cohort of young men aged 15–29 in the Americas represents only about half of 1 per cent (0.53 per cent) of the world's population (WHO 2002).

2 Having been a victim of violence (either in the home or outside the home) is strongly associated with being violent, but again the association is not absolute. Many boys and men, who have been victims of violence, abhor violence and use their experiences of witnessing or experiencing violence to rethink what it means to be a man. We found, in sample survey research with 750 men aged 15–60 in Rio de Janeiro, that 45 per cent of men reported having been victims of physical violence in their homes of origin (see Instituto Promundo and Instituto Noos 2003). In another study we carried out, we found that more than 22 per cent of boys aged 13–19 said they were victims of physical violence in their homes, compared to about 10 per cent in the case of girls. If serious physical violence is

more often carried out by the men – whether against men or women – physical violence is frequently part of the raising of boys.

3 With a few exceptions, young women in low-income settings where gangs are present are more likely to be indirectly involved as girlfriends of gang members, or in the administration or accounting of drug sales than in actual trafficking and carrying of weapons.

4 In early 2004, one of Rio's major newspapers compared deaths per day in US-occupied Iraq to the number of gang-related killings in Rio. On several days, there were more gang-related deaths in Rio.

6 No place at school

1 To give a sense of the socio-economic conditions in the community, according to 1990 census data, 64.7 per cent of the neighbourhood lived below the poverty line, compared to a citywide rate of 21.6 per cent. The adult unemployment rate in the area was 34.1 per cent, and 50.4 per cent of families received some public assistance.

2 Architecturally speaking, Chicago's large public high schools are impressive. They are usually red brick and white-trim facilities in the Prairie School style of architecture: they are more horizontal than vertical, following the long, flat lines of the Midwestern North American topography, and with long corridors and internal open spaces. They are typically built with lots of open space around them. In the case of this high school, there was an impressive courtyard in the middle of the school and high-ceiling hallways that extended for nearly a city block. The facilities were old but generally well maintained. The structure was impressive, but its dimensions were large. It was easy to feel small – symbolically and physically.

3 In spite of these messages in the school, during group sessions in the all guys' group, those young men who were sexually active were open about this and Mr Jones was open with them in return. He preferred that they kept their relationships non-sexual, but he understood their sexual desire and their right to make their own decision.

4 The source for these data is CESPI/USU and Promundo (2001). Among other issues, the survey involved asking young people about their participation in formal and informal youth groups and comparing the results by sex.

7 'If you don't work, you have to steal'

1 These data highlight the uneven nature of men's and women's economic marginalization and suggest the need to target specific groups of low-income men with employment and income-generation initiatives, for example low-income, unemployed fathers, as some programmes in Western Europe and North America have done (Arias 2001).

2 The informal sector is often but not always synonymous with lower wages. For some workers, the informal market has actually meant increased wages (Arias 2001).

3 While not the focus on this chapter, it is also worth noting that work that young men carry out is often dangerous or injurious to their health. According to official occupational health and safety data in Brazil, for 2002, young men aged 15–24 represented roughly one in five of all reported work-related accidents in Brazil. Taking into account the informal sector, there are an estimated 219,000 work-related accidents a year to young men (O Globo 2004b).

8 In the heat of the moment

1 This chapter has focused mainly on sexual and reproductive health needs. Nonetheless, research from various settings confirms similar trends with other health needs. In much of the world, boys are generally raised to be self-reliant, not to worry about their health and not to seek help when they face stress. Young men often see themselves as being invulnerable to illness or risk, and may just 'tough it out' when they are sick, or seek health services only as a last resort. In other cases, men may believe that clinics or hospitals are 'female' places (Barker 2000).

2 Testing and development is underway to produce microbicides that women can introduce into the vagina to prevent STIs, including HIV, which may be ready as early as 2009. Globally, there is a major initiative underway – called 'Three by five' – to make anti-retroviral medicines available to 3 million HIV-positive individuals around the world by 2005.

9 Learning to live with women, becoming fathers

1 In a study we carried out in Rio de Janeiro, 25.4 per cent of 749 men aged 15–60 had used physical violence at least once against an intimate female partner. Young men aged 20–24 had the highest rates of self-reported physical violence against women (in their current or most recent intimate relationship) than any other age range: 32 per cent of the young men reported that they had ever been physically violent with their current or most recent primary partner (Instituto Promundo and Instituto Noos 2003).

2 The consensus from research from Western Europe and North America is that when men (as social fathers or biological fathers) are involved in the lives of children, children benefit in terms of social and emotional development, often perform better in school and have healthier relationships as adults. However, this research also affirms that it appears that having multiple caregivers, or having a second caregiver to support a primary caregiver, is more important than the sex of the caregiver per se (NCOFF 2002; Lewis and Lamb 2003).

10 Dying to be men, living as men

1 Of course, young men in these settings are also affected by changes in gender norms at the broader societal level, such as campaigns or new laws related to gender-based violence.

2 Differences in attitudes were statistically significant in both communities. Changes in condom use and rates of STIs were only statistically significant in the community where group educational activities were combined with the Heat of the Moment campaign.

3 Several recent publications have described some of these emerging programme experiences (Interagency Gender Working Group 2003; Rivers and Aggleton 2002).

References

A Capital (2000) 'SIDA: A culpa é dos homens' [AIDS: Men are to blame], *A Capital*, 6 March.

Alan Guttmacher Institute (1998) *Facts in Brief: Teen Sex and Pregnancy*, New York: Alan Guttmacher Institute.

Alatorre, J. (2002) *Paternidad responsable en el istmo centroamericano* [Responsible Fatherhood in the Central American Isthmus], Mexico City: United Nations Economic Commission for Latin America and the Caribbean (CEPAL).

Anderson, E. (1990) *Streetwise: Race, Class and Change in an Urban Community*, Chicago: University of Chicago Press.

Aramburu, R. and Rodriguez, M. (1995) 'A puro valor mexicano: Conotaciones del uso del condón en hombres de la clase media en la Ciudad de México' [Pure Mexican force: Connotations of condom use in middle-class men in Mexico City], paper presented at the Coloquio Latinoamericano sobre Varones, Sexualidad y Reproducción, Zacatecas, Mexico, 17–18 November.

Archer, J. (1994) 'Violence between men', in J. Archer (ed.), *Male Violence*, London: Routledge.

Arias, O. (2001) 'Are men benefiting from the new economy? Male economic marginalization in Argentina, Brazil, and Costa Rica', Policy Research Working Paper no. 2740, Gender Sector Unit, World Bank Latin America and the Caribbean Region, Washington, DC: The World Bank.

Atkin, L. & Alatorre, J. (1991) 'The psychological meaning of pregnancy among adolescents in México City', paper presented at the Biennial Meeting of the Society for Research in Child Development, Seattle, WA, 18–20 April.

Ayres, R. (1998) *Crime and Violence as Development Issues in Latin America and the Caribbean*, Washington, DC: The World Bank.

Barcellos, C. (2003) *Abusado: O Dono do Morro Dona Marta* [Brat: The King of Dona Marta Hill], Rio de Janeiro: Editora Record.

Barker, G. (1998) 'Non-violent males in violent settings: An exploratory qualitative study of pro-social low income adolescent males in two Chicago (USA) neighborhoods', *Childhood: A Global Journal of Child Research*, 4: 437–61.

Barker, G. (2000a) *What about Boys? A Literature Review on the Health and Development of Adolescent Boys*, Geneva: World Health Organization.

Barker, G. (2000b) 'Gender equitable boys in a gender inequitable world: Reflections from qualitative research and programme development in Rio de Janeiro', *Sexual and Relationship Therapy*, 15/3: 263–82.

Barker, G., Nascimento, M., Segundo, M. and Pulerwitz, J. (2003) 'How do we know if men have changed? Promoting and measuring attitude change with young men', in S. Ruxton (ed.), *Lessons from Program H in Latin America, Gender Equality and Men*, Oxford: Oxfam.

Barker, G. & Loewenstein, I. (1997) 'Where the boys are: Attitudes related to masculinity, fatherhood and violence toward women among low income adolescent and young adult males in Rio de Janeiro, Brazil', *Youth and Society*, 29/2: 166–96.

Barker, G., Hall, C., Sharpe, J., Reiph-Arnell, J. and Boyce-Reid, K. (1995) 'Situation analysis of drug abuse among youth at risk in the Caribbean: A needs assessment of out-of-school youth in St. Vincent and the Grenadines, Trinidad and Tobago, St. Maarten and Jamaica', unpublished mimeo, Vienna: United Nations International Drug Control Programme.

Bell, C. and Jenkins, E. (1993) 'Community violence and children on Chicago's Southside', *Psychiatry*, 56: 46–54.

Bercovich, A., Dellasoppa, E. and Arriaga, E. (1998) '"J'adjuste, mais je ne corrige pas": Jovens, violencia e demografia no Brasil: Algumas reflexões a partir dos indicadores de violencia' [Youth, violence and demography in Brazil: Some reflections based on violence indicators], in Comissão Nacional de População e Desenvolvimento (CNPD) (eds), *Jovens Acontecendo na Trilha das Políticas Públicas* [Youth in the Path of Public Policy], Brasilia: CNPD.

Block, C.R. and Block, R. (1995) 'Street gang crime in Chicago', in M. Klein, C. Maxson and J. Miller (eds), *The Modern Gang Reader*, Los Angeles, CA: Roxbury.

Bourdieu, P. (1999) *A Dominação Masculina* [Male Domination], Rio de Janeiro: Bertrand Russell.

Brown, J. and Chevannes, B. (1998) *Why Man Stay So: An Examination of Gender Socialization in the Caribbean*, Kingston, Jamaica: University of the West Indies.

Brown, J., Newland, A., Anderson, P. and Chevannes, B. (1995) 'Caribbean fatherhood: Underresearched, misunderstood', Caribbean Child Development Centre and Department of Sociology and Social Work, University of the West Indies, Kingston, Jamaica, October.

Bruce, J., Lloyd, C. and Leonard, A. with Engle, P. and Duffy, N. (1995) *Families in Focus: New Perspectives on Mothers, Fathers and Children*, New York: Population Council.

CESPI/USU and Instituto Promundo (2001) *Children, Youth and their Developmental Supports: Strengthening Family and Community Supports for Children and Youth in Rio de Janeiro. Initial Results 2000–2001*, Rio de Janeiro, Brazil: CESPI/USU and Promundo.

Chant, S. and Gutmann, M. (2002) 'Men-streaming gender? Questions for gender and development policy in the twenty-first century', *Progress in Development Studies*, 2/4: 269–82.

Chevannes, B. (2001) *Learning to be a Man: Culture, Socialization and Gender Identity in Five Caribbean Communities*, Kingston, Jamaica: University of the West Indies Press.

Cincotta, R., Engelman, R. and Anastasion, D. (2003) *The Security Demographic: Population and Civil Conflict after the Cold War*. Washington DC: Population Action International.

Connell, R.W. (1994) *Masculinities*, Berkeley, CA: University of California Press.

Csikszentmihalyi, M. (2002) *Flow: The Classic Work on How to Achieve Happiness*, London: Rider.

De Keijzer, B. (1995) 'Masculinity as a risk factor', paper presented at the Coloquio Latinoamericano sobre 'Varones, Sexualidad y Reproduccion', Zacatecas, Mexico, 17–18 November.

Elliott, D. (1994) 'Serious violent offenders: Onset, developmental course and termination – The American Society of Criminology 1993 Presidential Address', *Criminology*, 32/1: 1–21.

Emler, N. and Reicher, S. (1995) *Adolescence and Delinquency: The Collective Management of Reputation*, Oxford: Blackwell.

Engle, P. (1997) 'The role of men in families: Achieving gender equity and supporting children', in C. Sweetman (ed.), *Men and Masculinity: Oxfam Focus on Gender*, Oxford: Oxfam.

Erikson, E. (1968) *Identity: Youth and Crisis*, New York: W.W. Norton.

Erikson, E. (1969) *Gandhi's Truth*, New York: W.W. Norton.

Ferguson, A.A. (2000) *Bad Boys: Public Schools in the Making of Black Masculinity*, Ann Arbor, MI: University of Michigan Press.

Fernandes, R.C. (2002) 'Educação de jovens em situação de risco: Dados do problema e ações da sociedade,' unpublished mimeo, Rio de Janeiro, Brazil: Viva Rio.

Figueroa, M. (1997) 'Gender privileging and socio-economic outcomes: The case of health and education in Jamaica', paper presented to the Ford Foundation Workshop on Family and the Quality of Gender Relations, Mona, Jamaica, 5–6 March.

Finger, W. (1998) 'Condom use increasing', *Network*, 18: 3 (Research Triangle Park, NC: Family Health International).

Fundação Mauricio Sirotsky Sobrinho, Fundação Odebrecht, Instituto Ayrton Senna, Instituto Credicard/Abrasso, Ministerio de Trabalho, UNICEF and Vitae (1997) *Educação Profissional de Adolescentes: Cadastro das Iniciativas Não-formais* [Vocational Training for Adolescents: A Review of Non-formal Initiatives], São Paulo, Brazil: The Authors.

Garcia-Hjarles, G. (2001) *Estudio aplicado de paternidad andina* [Applied Study of Andean Fatherhood], Lima, Peru: PMS Allin Tayta, Ministerio de Promoción de la Mujer y el Desarrollo Humano (PROMUDEH), Instituto Nacional de Bienestar Familiar (INABIF) and Ministerio de Educación (MINEDU).

Gardner, H. (1983) *Frames of mind: The theory of multiple intelligences*. New York: Basic Books.

Ghee, L.T. (2002) 'Youth and employment in the Asia-Pacific region: Prospects and challenges', paper presented at the Youth Employment Summit, Alexandria, Egypt, 7–11 September.

Gorgen, R., Yansane, M., Marx, M. and Millimounou, D. (1998) 'Sexual behaviors and attitudes among unmarried youths in Guinea', *International Family Planning Perspectives*, 24/2: 65–71.

Hamilton, T. and Associates (1995) *Final Report: Baseline Project for Uplifting Adolescents. Demographic and Ethnographic Analysis*. Unpublished document prepared for U.S. Agency for International Development–Jamaica. Kingston, Jamaica: Authors.

Heald, S. (1999) *Manhood and Morality: Sex, Violence and Ritual in Gisu Society*, London: Routledge.

Heise, L. (1994) 'Gender-based abuse: The global epidemic', *Caderno de Saúde Pública*, 10/1: 135–45.

Hopenhayn, M. (2002) 'Youth and employment in Latin America and the Caribbean: Problems, prospects, and options', paper presented at the Youth Employment Summit, Alexandria, Egypt, 7–11 September.

Horizons, 2004. Promoting Healthy Relationships and HIV/STI Prevention for Young Men: Positive findings from an intervention study in Brazil. Research update. April 2004. Washington DC. Horizons Program/Population Council.

Human Rights Watch/CLEEN (May 2002) 'The Bakassi Boys: The legitimization of murder and torture', *Human Rights Watch/CLEEN Reports*, 14/5 (whole issue).

Im-em, W. (1998) 'Sexual contact of Thai men before and after marriage', paper presented at the Seminar on Men, Family Formation and Reproduction, Buenos Aires, Argentina, 13–15 May.

Instituto Brasileiro de Geografia e Estadistica (IBGE) (1997) *Demographic Census of 1980, 1991/PNAD 1996*, Rio de Janeiro, Brazil: IBGE.

Instituto Brasileiro de Geografia e Estatistica (IBGE) (1998) *Pesquisa nacional por amostra de domicílios 1997* [National Household Survey 1997] (CD-Rom), Rio de Janeiro, Brazil: IBGE.

Instituto Brasileiro de Geografia e Estadistica (IBGE) (2004) *Censo demográfico – 2000* [Demographic Census 2002], Rio de Janeiro: IBGE. Available http://www.ibge.gov.br (accessed 4 March 2004).

Instituto Promundo and Instituto Noos (2003) *Men, Gender-based Violence and Sexual and Reproductive Health: A Study with Men in Rio de Janeiro/Brazil*, Rio de Janeiro: The Authors.

Instituto Promundo, ECOS, PAPAI, Salud y Género, International Planned Parenthood Federation/WHR and Pan American Health Organization (2002) *Project H: Manual Series for Working with Young Men in the Promotion of Health and Gender Equity*, São Paulo, Brazil: The Authors.

Interagency Gender Working Group/Subcommittee on Men and Reproductive Health (2003). Involving men to address gender inequities. Washington DC: Population Reference Bureau.

Jejeebhoy, S. (1996) 'Adolescent sexual and reproductive behavior: A review of evidence from India', ICRW Working Paper no. 3, Washington, DC: International Center for Research on Women.

Jezl, D., Molidor, C. and Wright, T. (1996) 'Physical, sexual and psychological abuse in high school dating relationships: Prevalence rates and self-esteem issues', *Child and Adolescent Social Work Journal*, 13/1: 69–87.

Kaufman, M. (1993) *Cracking the Armour: Power, Pain and the Lives of Men*, Toronto: Viking.

Levinson, D. (1989) *Violence in Cross-cultural Perspective*, Newbury Park, CA: Sage.

Lewis, C. and Lamb, M. (2003) 'Fathers: The research perspective', draft document prepared for the International Fatherhood Summit, Oxford, UK, February.

Linhales Barker, S. (1995) 'The disguised: A study on the production of subjectivity among low income adolescents in a favela in Rio de Janeiro', unpublished master's thesis, State University of Rio de Janeiro, Brazil.

Lyra, J. (1998) 'Paternidade adolescente: Da investigação a intervenção' [Adolescent fatherhood: From research to intervention], in M. Arilha, S. Ridenti and B. Medrado (eds) *Homens e Masculinidades: Outras Palavras* [Men and Masculinities: Other Words], São Paulo, Brazil: ECOS and Editora 34.

McAlister, A. (1998) *La violencia juvenil en las Americas: Estudios innovadores de investigacion, diagnostico y prevención* [Youth Violence in the Americas: Innovative Studies, Diagnosis and Prevention], Washington, DC: Pan American Health Organization.

Magdol, L., Moffitt, T., Caspi, A., Newman, D., Fagan, J. and Silva, P. (1997) 'Gender differences in partner violence in a birth cohort of 21-year-olds: Bridging the gap between clinical and epidemiological approaches', *Journal of Consulting and Clinical Psychology*, 65/1: 68–78.

Majors, R. and Billson, J.M. (1993) *Cool Pose: The Dilemmas of Black Manhood in America*, New York: Touchstone.

Marsiglio, W. (1988) 'Adolescent male sexuality and heterosexual masculinity: A conceptual model and review', *Journal of Adolescent Research*, 3/3–4: 285–303.

Mead, M. (1949) *Male and Female*, New York: William Morrow.

Mesquida, C. and Wiener, N. (1999) *Male age composition and severity of conflicts*. Politics and Life Sciences, 18(2) 181–189.

Michailof, S., Kostner, M. and Devictor, X. (2002) *Post-Conflict Recovery in Africa: An agenda for the Africa region*. Africa Region Working Paper Series No.30, April 2002. Washington DC: The World Bank.

Moser, C. and Van Bronkhorst, B. (1999) 'Youth violence in Latin America and the Caribbean: Costs, causes, and interventions', LCR Sustainable Development Working Paper no. 3, Urban Peace Program Series, Washington, DC: The World Bank.

National Center for Health Statistics (NCHS) (2003) *Homicide*, Hyattsville, MD: NCHS. Available http//www.cdc.gov/nchs/homicide.htm (accessed 22 September 2003).

National Center on Fathers and Families (NCOFF) (2002) *The Fathering Indicators Framework: A Tool for Quantitative and Qualitative Analysis*, Philadelphia, PA: NCOFF.

Necchi, S. and Schufer, M. (1998) *Adolescente varón: Iniciación sexual y conducta reproductiva* [The Adolescent Male: Sexual Initiation and Reproductive Behavior], Buenos Aires, Argentina: Programa de Adolescência, Hospital de Clínicas, Universidad de Buenos Aires/OMS/CONICET.

New York Times (2003) 'Japan's new homeless, there's disdain and danger', *New York Times*, 17 December.

Nolasco, S. (1993) *O Mito da Masculinidade* [The Myth of Masculinity], Rio de Janeiro, Brazil: Rocco.

O Globo (2002a) 'Jovens longe da escola ficam mais perto do trafico' [Youth out of school are 'in' with gangs], *O Globo*, 29 September.

O Globo (2002b) 'O primeiro e ultimo emprego: Trafico oferece mais trabalho a jovens de 15 a 17 anos do que o mercado formal' [The first and last job: Drug trafficking offers more jobs to youth 15 to 17 years old than the formal job market], 8 December.

O Globo (2002c) 'UNICEF: educação dos jovens no país é alarmante' [UNICEF: Educational status of youth in country is alarming], 12 December.

O Globo (2003) 'Número de inscrições para gari bate recorde' [Number of applications for garbage collector beats record], 26 June.

O Globo (2004a) 'Cariocas constroem "bunkers" dentro de casa' [Residents of Rio
de Janeiro construct 'bunkers' in their houses], *O Globo*, 18 January.

O Globo (2004b) 'Jovens de até 24 anos sofrem mais acidentes' [Youth under age
24 suffer more accidents], 14 March.

O Globo (2004c) 'População do país vai parar de crescer em 2062' [Population will
stop growing in 2062], 31 August.

Okojie, C. (2003) Employment Creation for Youth in Africa: The Gender
Dimension. Paper presented at Jobs for Youth: National Strategies for
Employment Promotion, 15–16 June. Geneva, Switzerland.

Pan American Health Organization, World Health Organization and Population
Reference Bureau (2003) *Gender, health, and development in the Americas:*
2003, Washington, DC: PAHO, WHO and PRB.

Panos Institute (1998) 'AIDS and men: Old problem, new angle', Panos HIV/AIDS
Briefing no. 6, London: Panos.

Pollack, W. (1998) *Real Boys: Rescuing our Sons from the Myths of Boyhood*, New
York: Random House.

Ribeiro, R. & Saboia, A. (1994) 'Children in Brazil: Legislation and citizenship', in
I. Rizzini (ed.), *Children in Brazil Today: A Challenge for the Third Millennium*,
Rio de Janeiro, Brazil: Editora Universidade Santa Úrsula.

Rivers, K. and Aggleton, P. (2002) *Working with Young Men to Promote Sexual and*
Reproductive Health. London: Safe Passages to Adulthood.

Rodgers, D. (1999) 'Youth gangs and violence in Latin America and the Caribbean:
A literature survey', LCR Sustainable Development Working Paper no. 4, Urban
Peace Program Series, Washington, DC: The World Bank.

Sampson, R.J. & Laub, J.H. (1993) *Crime in the Making: Pathways and Turning*
Points through Life, Cambridge, MA: Harvard University Press.

Schwartz, G. (1987) *Beyond Conformity or Rebellion: Youth and Authority in*
America, Chicago, IL: University of Chicago Press.

Senderowitz, J. (1995) 'Adolescent health: Reassessing the passage to adulthood',
World Bank Discussion Paper no. 272, Washington, DC: The World Bank.

Shweder, R. (2003) *Why do Men Barbecue? Recipes for Cultural Psychology*,
Cambridge, MA: Harvard University Press.

Silva, E. (1995) 'O movimento comunitário de Nova Holanda: Na busca do
encontro entre o político e o pedagógico' [The community movement in Nova
Holanda: Searching for the meeting of the political and the pedagogical],
unpublished master's thesis, Pontifica Universidade Catolica do Rio de Janeiro,
Brazil.

Singh, S., Wulf, D., Samara, R. and Cuca, P. (2000) 'Gender differences in the timing of first intercourse: Data from 14 countries', *International Family Planning*
Perspectives, 26/1: 21–8, 43.

Sonenstein, F., Pleck, J. and Ku, L. (1995) *Why Young Men don't Use Condoms:*
Factors Related to the Consistency of Utilization, Washington, DC: The Urban
Institute.

Souza e Silva, J. (2003) *Por que uns e não Outros? Caminhada de Jovens Pobres*
para a Universidade [Why Some and not Others? Pathways of Poor Youth to
University], Rio de Janeiro: 7Letras.

Souza e Silva, J. & Urani, A. (2002) 'Situation of children in drug trafficking: A rapid assessment', Investigating the Worst Forms of Child Labor, no. 20, Brazil, Geneva: International Programme on the Elimination of Child Labour (IPEC), ILO.

Tauchen, H., Witte, A.D. and Long, S.K. (1991) 'Domestic violence: A nonrandom affair', *International Economic Review*, 32: 491–511.

Taylor, R. (1991) 'Poverty and adolescent black males: The subculture of disengagement', in P. Edelman and J. Ladner (eds) *Adolescence and Poverty: Challenge for the 1990s*, Washington, DC: Center for National Policy Press.

Teixeira, H. (1997) 'O jovem no mercado de trabalho', *Revista Brasileira de Educação*, Numero especial, Juventude e Contemporaneidade [Special issue, Contemporary Youth], 5–6: 15–22.

United Nations (1995) The World's Women 1995: Trends and Statistics. New York: United Nations.

UNAIDS (1999) *Report on the Global HIV/AIDS Epidemic*, Geneva: UNAIDS. Available http://www.unaids.org (accessed 1 March, 2002)

UNESCO (2002) *Education for All Global Monitoring Report: Is the World on Track?* Montreal: UNESCO Institute for Statistics.

UNFPA (2003) *State of the World Population 2003*, New York: UNFPA.

UNICEF (2004) *Situação Mundial da Infancia 2004* [The State of the World's Children 2004], New York: UNICEF.

US Department of Health and Human Services (1991) *Vol. 2, Part A 'Mortality'*, Tables 1–9, 'Death Rates for 72 Selected Caused by 5-Year Age Groups, Race and Sex, U.S. 1988', Washington, DC: US DHHS.

Urdal, H. (2002). The Devil in the Demographics: How Youth Bulges Influence the Risk of Domestic Armed Conflict, 1950–2000. Paper presented at the International Studies Association 43rd Annual Convention, New Orleans LA, 24–27 March 2002.

Verhey, B. (2001) 'Child soldiers: Preventing, demobilizing and reintegrating', World Bank Africa Region Working Paper Series no. 23, Washington, DC: The World Bank.

Wacquant, L. (2001) *As Prisões da Miséria* [The Prisons of Misery], Rio de Janeiro, Brazil: Jorge Zahar Editor.

Wilson, W.J. (1996) *When Work Disappears: The World of the New Urban Poor*, New York: Vintage.

World Bank (1996) *Report on Human Development in Brazil*, Washington, DC: The World Bank.

World Bank (1997) *World Development Report 1997: The State of a Changing World*, New York: Oxford University Press.

World Health Organization (1995) *Human Reproduction Programme Annual Technical Report 1995: Executive Summary*, Geneva: WHO.

World Health Organization (2002) *World Report on Violence and Health*, Geneva: WHO.

Wyss, B. (1995) 'Gender and economic support of Jamaican households: Implications for children's living standards', doctoral dissertation, University of Massachusetts, Amherst.

Zaluar, A. (1994) 'Gangsters and remote-control juvenile delinquents: Youth and crime', in I. Rizzini (ed.), *Children in Brazil Today: A Challenge for the Third Millennium*, Rio de Janeiro, Brazil: Editora Universitaria Santa Ursula.

Index

Note: The index covers the main text, notes and appendix

abortion, selective 1
Abusado (Barcellos) 60
Africa: armed conflict 61–2;
  employment 103; rituals of manhood
  16–17; sexual relationships 117–18,
  125
African American youth: education 90,
  93–6; and law enforcement 50, 51;
  male identity 20–1; social exclusion
  42–4, 55
African Brazilian (*Afro-brasileiro*) 171
African National Congress (ANC) 2,
  156
Afro-brasileiro 171
AIDS, *see* HIV/AIDS
Al hajis 49
ANC, *see* African National Congress
Anderson, Elijah 42
anger 48–9, 110
anger control 149
Argentina 124
armed groups 61–2, 70
Asia, Southern 1, 128, 135
attention deficit problems 66
attitudes, towards young women
  119–24, 131–3
awareness 9–10: emotional 149

baile funk (funk dances) 126–8
Bakassi Boys 62–3
banana cropping 105
bandido identity 69, 71
Barcellos, C. 60
behavioural problems 66
bonde 56–7
Bourdieu, P. 18
'boy's code' (Pollack) 18
brands, marketing 54–5

Brazil: arrests of young men 4–5;
  deaths of young men 2–3; definitions
  of manhood 19; drug-trafficking
  gangs 70; education 87, 97;
  employment 102–3, 106, 108; law
  enforcement 51–2; military service
  111; poverty 39–40; research
  background and methodology
  160–4; sexual relationships of young
  men 119; social exclusion 56–7;
  staying out of gangs 81; violence
  against women 138, 141
Byrne, David 25

Canada 141
Caribbean: economic difficulties 41–2;
  education 86, 91; employment 104,
  105–7; HIV/AIDS 128; law
  enforcement 49–50; male-female
  relationships 123–4; research
  background and methodology 158;
  value of education 97; violence 61,
  137
case studies: João 28–35, 66, 122–3,
  144, 150; Murilo 67–70, 82
Central America, migrants 43–4
Chicago US: definitions of manhood
  19–20; education 92, 93–6, 172;
  employment 111; gangs 70, 171,
  staying out of 74–6, 81; Hispanic
  youth 43–4, 55–6, 77–8, 171; law
  enforcement 50–1, 51; male-female
  relationships 119–20, 125, 126;
  research background and
  methodology 159–60; social
  exclusion 42–4; violence, against
  women 140–1; violence, impacts of
  77–8

childbearing: early 39, 94, 143; and
 male employment 111–12
childhood, predictors of violent
 behaviour 63
children: care 104, 148; soldiers 62;
 witnessing of domestic violence
 139–40, 141
chlamydia infections 129
Christian-Muslim conflict, Nigeria 45,
 62, 78–81
Cidade de Deus (Lin) 59–60
Cincotta, R. 5
circumcision, male 17, 170
civil service jobs, Nigeria 102–3,
 109–10, 121
classism 27, 46–7
code of manhood 17–18
Colombia 15–16, 22, 27, 60, 137
comandos 2, 28, 36–9, 68, 69, 71–2;
 impacts of violence 77; presumed
 connections with 48, 65–6
common entrance examinations,
 Caribbean 91
communas 16
communication, social exclusion 154–5
community-based youth programmes
 99–100
condom use 119, 128–30, 167, 173
conflict: armed 61–2; religious groups
 45, 62, 78–81
Connell, R.W. 7
Conscientizing Male Adolescents,
 Nigeria 132
consumerism 40, 54–5
contraceptive use 119, 128–30
'cool pose' 43
critical reflection 131–2, 148, 152, 153
Csikszentmihalyi, Mihaly 99
cultures: definitions of manhood
 19–22; role of 55; and violence
 against women 139

dances, funk, Brazil 126–8
de Souza e Silva, Jailson 39–40
'dead-beat' dads 113
death, causes in young men 1, 2, *see
 also* homicides
decision-making 10
delinquency, and violence 65
demographic factors 5–6, 11, 102
development: adolescent 170;
 neurological 9–10; violence as
 phenomenon of 11

dialogues, internal 20, 57
discrimination 46–9
diversity, in young men's behaviours
 117, 118, 145
DJs 119–20
dress 48
drug trafficking 105, 106, 108; gangs
 28, 31, 36–9, 70; income from 72
drug use 33–4

economic factors 39, 40, 41–2, 113–14
education: boy enrolment and drop-out
 rates 84–6, 87–93; 'feminine' style of
 90; girls 84, 87; sex 130–1; South
 Side of Chicago 93–6; traditional/
 rigid systems 91, *see also* schools
educational attainment 86–7; and
 employment prospects 96–8; Maré
 favela 35, 39–40; and marriage 136
El Salvador 63
elders, *see* older men
elites 110
emotional intelligence 149
employment: Brazil 106–7; Caribbean
 41–2, 105–7; competition with
 education 85–6, 87; competition for
 44–5, 102–3; economic factors 41–2,
 113–14; and fatherhood 142, 144;
 gang involvement 72, 73–4; health
 and safety 172; informal sector
 30–1, 113–14, 144, 172; meaning
 for young men 19, 72–3, 102, 103,
 104, 108–9, 136; military service
 111; Nigeria 45–6, 102–3, 109–10;
 pressure to work 107–11; and sexual
 relationships 111–13; skills 113–16;
 value of education for 96–8; women
 44–5, 103, 104, 107, 121–2, *see also*
 unemployment
employment training programmes 106,
 116
Engender Health 156
Erikson, Erik 90, 155, 157, 170
Escobar, Carlos 15, 16
ethnicity, and violence 45, 78–81
evangelical churches 48

'face', loss of 43
families: formation and employment
 111–13; headed by women 53–4;
 influential members 54, 146; and
 school drop-outs 91; support of
 resistance to norms 146; and youth
 gang involvement 73, 75

fatherhood 19–20, 29, 33, 173; and employment 111–13; young men 142–4

fathers: absence from households 53–4; 'dead-beat' dads 113; involvement in child's upbringing 173; relationships with children 68

favelado 47

favelas, Brazil 2: brand marketing 54–5; classism 47; drug trafficking 70; employment 30–1; Maré 35–9; sexual relationships 126–8; social exclusion 56–7; violence 27, 69, 171

fear, of gang-related violence 76

Ferguson, A.A. 42

fertility, pressure to prove 135–6, 143

films 18, 59–60

fishing 105–6

'flow' 99

football 13–14

frustration 10

gangbanger 2

gangs 2; anti-school 98–9; drug-trafficking 28, 31, 36–9, 70; homicides 63; and male identity 20–1, 83; and male-female relationships 32–3, 71–2, 172; prevalence of 70; reasons for joining 40, 57, 70–4, 82–3, 98–9; reasons for staying out of 31–3, 74–6, 81–2, 147, 149–50

Gardner, Howard 149

gender 7–8; and education 3; 'matrix' 16–19, 32–3

gender equity 131–3, 147–8; initiatives 151–3

gender norms 17–19, 119–24; changes 151–4, 173; resistance to 23–4

gender stereotypes 99

'gender studies' 7, 112

Gender-Equitable in Men (GEM) Scale 153, 166–7, 170

girls: early childbearing 39, 94, 143; education 3, 84, 87; and gang members 32–3, 71–2, 172; involved in violence 61; 'missing' 1; socialization 88, 100

Global Emergency AIDS Act (US) 4

globalization 40

grandmothers 54

Grenadines 49

Guinea 125

habitus 18

'harlots' 120

health services 173

'hidden ones' 78

'hippy' identity 12, 13

Hispanic youth, US 43–4, 55–6, 77–8, 171

HIV/AIDS 3–4, 128–9; condom use 128–30; Joint United Nations Programme 4; prevention 4, 131, 173; rates of infection 128; support and prevention programmes 155–6; transmission 3–4, 6, 117, 118; treatment 173; women 150–1

homicides 1, 171; gang-related 38, 63; rates of 1, 60–1; schools 14–15; young women 171

homosexual relationships 118

Honduras 104

'hood rats' 120

hope 155–7

Horizons Program 153

Houston, Texas 12–13

identity, *see* male identity

idle time 42, 46

illiteracy 86, 87

imagination, development 9–10

imprisonment 4–5, 50

In the Heat of the Moment Campaign, Brazil 141

Inthaka Freedom Party, South Africa 156

income: and fatherhood 142; from drug-trafficking 72; inequality 27, 63–4; and relationships 136; value of education for 96–8; womens' 112–13

India 1, 135

inequality 27, 63–4

infanticide, female 1

infidelity, sexual 138

initiatives: AIDS prevention 4, 131; fatherhood 142–3; prevention of violence against women 141; women's employment 113

Instituto Promundo, Brazil 131, 153

Integrated Centres for Primary Education (CIEPs) 36

internal dialogues 20, 57

International Labour Office (ILO) 70, 71–2, 103

Jamaica 49, 86, 105, 106
Jihad! 80
João 28–35, 66, 122–3, 144, 150
jobs, *see* employment
'jock' identity 13–14
Joint United Nations Programme on
    HIV/AIDS 4
justice systems 49–53

'kicker' identity 12, 13, 22
killings, by police 15–16, 26, *see also*
    homicides
knives, carrying of 61

labelling, of young men 48, 57, 65–6,
    68, 69, 89, 96
Lahore, Pakistan 125, 127
Latin America: deaths of young men 1;
    education 87; youth unemployment
    104, *see also named countries*
law enforcement 49–53
learned behaviours 65, 139–40
Liberia 62
'limin' 42
Lin, Paulo 59–60
literacy 86, 87
literature 59–60

machismo 122
male circumcision, Africa 17, 170
male identity: alternatives to norms
    31–3; 'cool pose' 43; development
    170; and employment 19, 72–3, 102,
    103, 104; and gang membership
    20–1, 71, 82–3; in schools 12–14;
    and sexual relationships 124–6;
    struggles with 21–2; and violence 59,
    66–7, 69, 71, *see also* manhood
male-female relationships: and
    employment 43, 111–13; gang
    members 32–3, 71–2, 172; positive
    123–4; resistance to gender norms
    146–7; stress in 136–41; violence
    119, 123, *see also* mothers; sexual
    relationships
manhood: cultural definitions of
    19–22; hierarchies 9; rites of passage
    16–18; and sexual relationships 124,
    see also male identity
Maré *favela*, Brazil 28, 35–9, 47, 48, 56
marijuana 106
marketing, consumer goods 40, 54–5
Marley, Bob 98

marriage: arranged/forced 135; and
    educational attainment 136; gang
    members 71–2; pressure on young
    men 135–6
The Matrix 18
media 24, 37, 38
Men Can Stop Rape, US 141
mental hospitals 50
metacognitive skills 34, 149
Mexico 43–4
middle classes: discrimination of youth
    30, 46–7; fears of violence 60; in
    violence 83; young men's anger
    towards 48–9
migrants 43–4
migration 104
military: careers/service 111;
    harassment of youth 110
'missing' women and girls 1
'missing' young men 1
money, *see* income
mothers: heading households 53–4;
    relationships with children 67
movies 18, 59–60
Murilo 67–70, 82, 122, 132
music, involvement in 55, 75–6
Muslim-Christian conflict, Nigeria 45,
    62, 78–81

'nerd' identity 13
New Zealand 137
newspapers 38
Nicaragua 63, 137
Nigeria: armed groups 62–3, 70;
    definitions of manhood 19;
    employment 45–6, 102–3, 109–10;
    law enforcement 51; marriages 135;
    Muslim-Christian conflict 45, 62,
    78–81; research background and
    methodology 168–9; resistance to
    gender norms 24; social exclusion
    44–6; young men's views of women
    120–1
Nike shoes 54–5
norms, gender 17–19, 119–24
Nova Holanda, Rio de Janeiro Brazil
    35–9, 56–7

occupational health and safety 172
older men 20; absence from households
    53–4; anger of young men towards
    110; Nigeria 49; relationships with
    women 118, 137; as role models 32

Once in a Lifetime (Talking Heads) 25
Once Upon a Boy 165

pain, enduring/inflicting 17
Pakistan 124–5, 127
Panos Institute 118
parents: protection of children from
    violence 64; relationships with
    children 67–8, 69
'patriarchal dividend' 7
peer groups: anti-school 90, 91; pro-
    social 56–7; and school troubles 89;
    and sexual experiences 125; and
    violence 65, 66–7, 69
Peru 104
police 37, 49–53; brutality 38, 51–2;
    harassment of young men 31, 47;
    killings 15–16, 26
Pollack, W. 18
population structure 5–6, 11, 102
poverty 27, 39–40, 88; and violence
    63–4, *see also* income, inequality
power, and violence 66
powerlessness 57, 66
prisons 4–5, 50
Program H, Brazil, Mexico 132,
    151–3, 164–8
protection: gangs 73; peer groups 56–7
puberty 130
punitive policies 4–5

racism 27, 47–9, 90
rap music 55
reflective abilities 131–2, 148, 152, 153
relationships: with parents 67–8, 69,
    see also male-female relationships
religion 147
religious conflict 45, 62, 78–81
religious groups 48, 57, 81
reputations, and male identity 13
research sites and methodologies
    158–64
resistance 146–50; promotion of
    151–4; to gang membership 31–4; to
    gender norms 23–4, 146–50
responsibility 144
Rio de Janeiro: drug-trafficking gangs
    31, 70; educational attainment 87;
    employment 106–7, 108; gangs,
    staying out of 31–3, 75; law
    enforcement 52; research
    background and methodology

160–4; sexual relationships of young
    men 119, 126–8; violence, costs of
    61, gang-related 172, limits of 26–8,
    see also favelas
rituals, passage to manhood 16–18
role models 6, 32; work 114–15
'Romeo' identity, US 16–17, 94

St Vincent 49, 105–6
schools: buildings 36, 172; choice of
    male identity 12–14, 22; engaging
    boys in 98–9; expulsions 68, 95;
    'failed' students 91–2; gender issues
    3; labelling of young men 65–6, 68,
    89, 96; male peer groups 89–90;
    South Side of Chicago 93–6; support
    and discussion groups 93–6, 172;
    violence 14–15, 37, 61, *see also*
    education; educational attainment;
    teachers
self-reflection 131–2, 148, 152, 153
sex: age of first 3, 124; before marriage
    119; condom use 119, 128–30;
    education 95, 130–1; *favelas* 126–8;
    and HIV/AIDS transmission 3–4;
    meaning to young men 124–6;
    ritualized 17
sexual abuse 119
sexual harassment 44, 92–3, 103,
    121–2
sexual infidelity 138
sexual relationships: formation of
    stable 134–6; reasons for 117; same
    sex 118; what boys want to know
    130–1; young men's attitudes
    119–24, *see also* male-female
    relationships
sexually-transmitted infections (STIs)
    118; prevention 173; rates of 128,
    129, *see also* HIV/AIDS
Sierra Leone 62
social exclusion 6, 27–8; brand
    marketing 54–5; Caribbean 41–2;
    coping with 55–7; and law
    enforcement 49–53; living with
    30–1; Nigeria 44–6; racial and class
    discrimination 46–9; and resistance
    to violence 33–5; silence of young
    men 154–5; United States 42–4
social habitus 18
social inequalities 10
social institutions: breakdown 64, *see
    also* families; schools

social skills 114–16
socialization 100; gender differences
    88–9; girls 88, 100
South Africa 2, 62; HIV/AIDS 155–6;
    violence 61, 62, 63, 70, 156–7
South Asia 1, 128, 135
sports 13–14, 99
sports groups 57
status, gang membership 40, 72–3
stereotypes 48, 65–6, 69, 89, 99; male
    sexual 117; psychological impacts
    57–8; violent 65–6; women 113;
    young fathers 142
STIs, see sexually-transmitted infections
stress: and employment 107–11; male-
    female relationships 123, 136–41;
    parents/families 64
structural violence 27, 57
sub-Saharan Africa 103; AIDS 128
support groups, schools 93–6, 172

teachers: labelling of young men 65–6,
    68, 89, 96; women 89, 90, 92
training programmes 106, 116
travel, outside local communities 46–8
Trinidad and Tobago 42, 86

Uganda 17, 117–18, 170
unemployment: and crime 109; rates of
    163–4, see also employment
United Nations Educational, Scientific
    and Cultural Organization
    (UNESCO) 3
United Nations Population Fund
    (UNFPA) 3, 10
United in Peace, Brazil 56
United States: gang-related violence 63;
    homicide rate 16; social exclusion of
    young men 42–4; violence against
    women 137, 138, see also Chicago

variation, young men's behaviours 117,
    118, 145
vigilante groups 62–3
violence: against women 2, 119, 123,
    137–41, 151, 171, 173; case study
    (Murilo) 67–70, 82; as
    developmental phenomenon 11;

drug-related 31; and ethnicity
    78–81; gang-related 38, 63, 76, 172;
    girls involved in 61; in the home
    171; as learned behaviours 65,
    139–40; limits to 26–7; and male
    identity 66–7; non-fatal 61; personal
    impacts 76–8, 146; portrayal in films
    and literature 59–60; and power 66;
    prevalence rates 60–1; public costs
    61; rejection/resistance 148–9;
    schools 37; structural 27, 57;
    theories on causation 63–7; victims
    171; witnessing of 139–40, 141, 155
voices of resistance 23–4, 145, 146–50

Wacquant, L. 5
'warrior ethos' 69
West Africa 125
whaling 105–6
White Ribbon Campaign 141
'whores' 120
Wilson, W.J. 42
women: attitudes of young men
    towards 119–24; early childbearing
    143; education 3; employment 44–5,
    103, 104, 107, 112–13, 121–2; and
    gang members 32–3, 72; genital
    cutting 170; heading households
    53–4; HIV/AIDS 150–1; income of
    112–13; involved in violence 61;
    'missing' 1; role in making of men
    150–1; sexual harassment 44,
    121–2; social exclusion 57; STIs
    128; teachers 89, 90, 92; violence
    against 2, 119, 123, 137–41, 151,
    173, see also girls
work, see employment
World Bank 5, 39
World Health Organization (WHO) 3,
    61, 62, 63, 135

youth: age boundaries 9; population
    boom 5–6, 11, 102
youth programmes 99–100, 116

Zaluar, Alba 69, 71
zero tolerance policies 5, 66, 95